Cambridge Level 3 Advanced National

HEALTH & SOCIAL CARE (AAQ)

Revision Guide

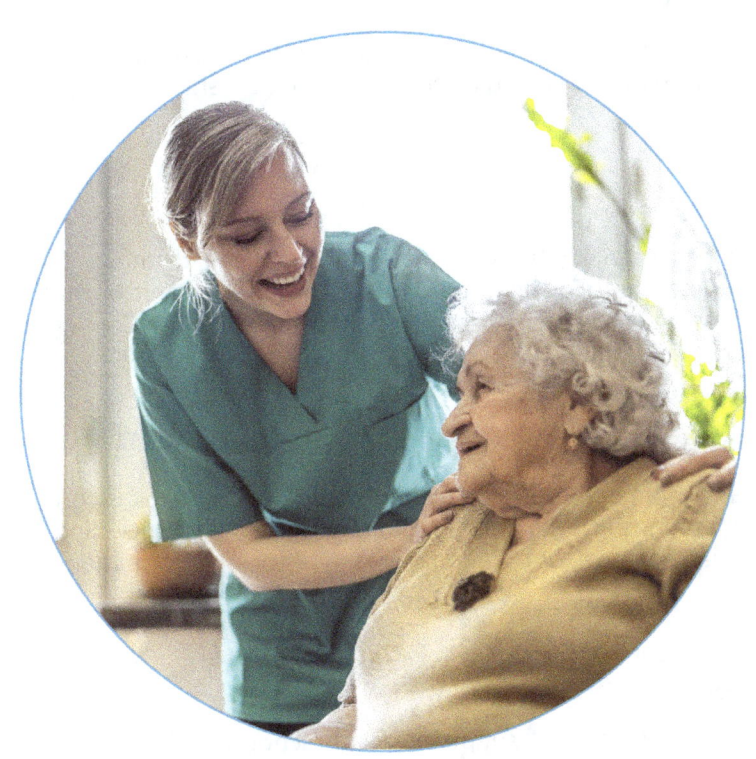

Alison Lockyer

eboru

The publisher gratefully acknowledges the permission of copyright holders to reproduce copyright material.

Page 16: The Eatwell Guide is subject to Crown copyright protection, which is covered by an Open Government Licence. Source: OHID in association with the Welsh government, Food Standards Scotland and the Food Standards Agency in Northern Ireland.

Please see the remaining photo credits at: www.eboru.com/Cambridge-HSC-RG-PhotoCredits

Cover image: © pikselstock/Shutterstock

Every effort has been made to trace copyright holders and to obtain their permission for the use of copyright material. The publisher will be glad to make arrangements with any copyright holder it has not been possible to contact.

Copyright © 2025 Alison Lockyer

All rights reserved. No part of this publication may be reproduced, distributed, or transmitted in any form or by any means, including photocopying, recording, or other electronic or mechanical methods, without the prior written permission of the publisher, or under licence from the Copyright Licensing Agency. See www.cla.co.uk for more details.

First edition 2025. Impression 10 9 8 7 6 5 4 3 2 1

ISBN: 978-1-917048-04-0

Whilst every effort has been made to ensure all information in this book is correct, the publisher shall not be liable for any loss of profit or any other commercial damages, including but not limited to special, incidental, consequential, personal, or other damages, due to any information or advice contained in this book.

Ordering Information

Special discounts are available for class set purchases by schools, colleges and others. For details, contact the publisher at: orders@eboru.com

Trade orders: copies of this book are available through the normal wholesalers. For any queries please contact: orders@eboru.com

www.eboru.com

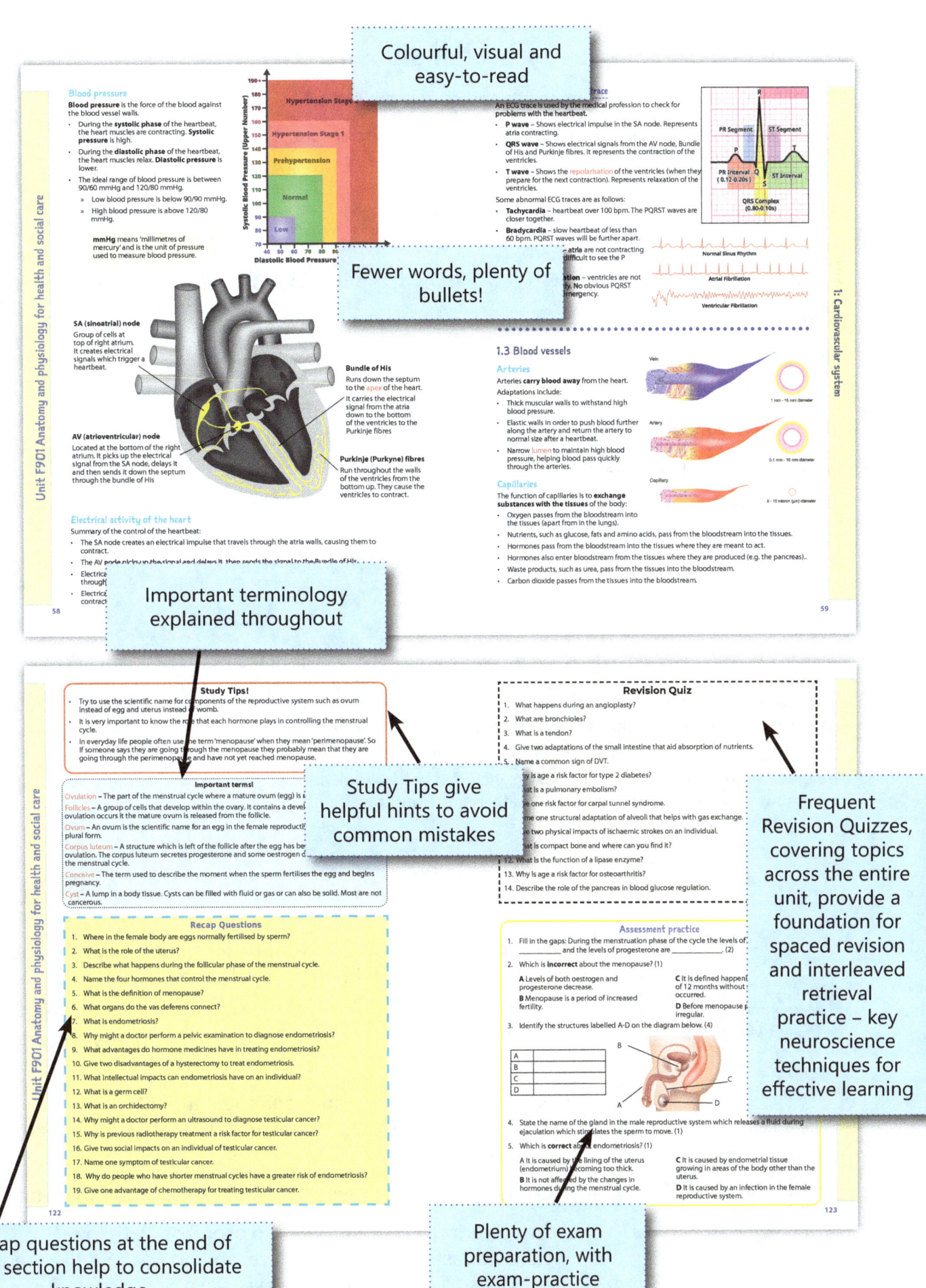

Contents

Unit F090: Principles of health and social care — 5

1: Equality, diversity, and rights in health and social care settings — 7
2: Managing hazards, health and safety in health and social care settings — 23
3: Legislation in health and social care settings — 34
4: Best practice in health and social care settings — 45

Unit F091: Anatomy and physiology for health and social care — 55

1: Cardiovascular system — 55
2: Respiratory system — 69
3: Digestive system — 79
4: Musculoskeletal system — 89
5: Control and regulatory systems — 101
6: Reproductive system — 114

Answers are available at: www.eboru.com/Cambridge-HSC-RG-Answers

---

While this book is designed to help and support teachers and learners throughout the course the only official source of information about the qualification is the qualification specification and associated assessment guidance, published by the awarding organisation. Teachers and students should always refer to the specification and sample assessment material for definitive information about all aspects of this qualification. Specifications are also updated from time to time.

The practice questions, marks and answers included in this book are designed to help learners develop their knowledge, skills, understanding and technique but they do not replicate real examination papers, assessments or mark schemes.

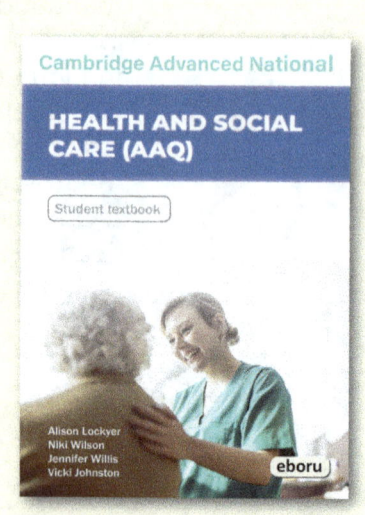

ISBN: 978-0-9929002-9-8

Covering **all units**, this student book for the new Cambridge Advanced National Health and Social Care (AAQ) is your perfect companion!

- Visual: Colourful and attractive design, with less text and more images
- Engaging: Written in language that students can understand, with keyword boxes for unfamiliar words on each spread
- Comprehensive: Covers all mandatory and optional units
- Empowering: Helps students to progress, with low-stakes questions for frequent recap and Case Studies and Activities to develop higher-level skills

Unit F090: Principles of health and social care

Introduction

This unit relates to both health and social care settings.

- **Health care settings** focus on illness and injury and include settings that diagnose, treat and manage medical conditions.
- **Social care settings** support people with daily living activities where they are struggling due to age, disability or long-term conditions.
- The specific health and social care settings that your exam might refer to are shown below.

Health care settings

Setting	What it does
Dental practice	Looks after oral health including check-ups, fillings and tooth extractions. They also provide advice on how to look after oral health.
GP surgery/ health centre	Primary care centres for non-emergency medical issues. They are the first point of contact between a patient and the health service and can refer individuals to specialists for diagnosis and treatment. They help individuals manage long-term conditions.
Hospice	Provide support to people who are at the end of their life (known as palliative or end-of-life care). Services can be in a hospice, within the person's own home or elsewhere.
Hospital	Secondary care setting which provides a range of health services including surgery, specialist treatments and emergency care.
Mobile health screening unit	Specialist vehicles that spend time in different locations, such as supermarket car parks, in order to be more accessible. They screen for different conditions, such as breast cancer.
Nursing home	A care home providing long-term care to people who are no longer able to be looked after at home. They are staffed by both care assistants and registered nurses.
Opticians	Support people with eye health and vision by providing eye tests, prescribing glasses and contact lenses and monitoring eye health.
Pharmacy	Provide medicine prescribed by medical professionals and also over-the-counter medicine. They also provide services like some vaccinations, blood pressure checks and offer advice on some conditions.
Walk-in centre	Treat minor illnesses and injuries without the need for an appointment.

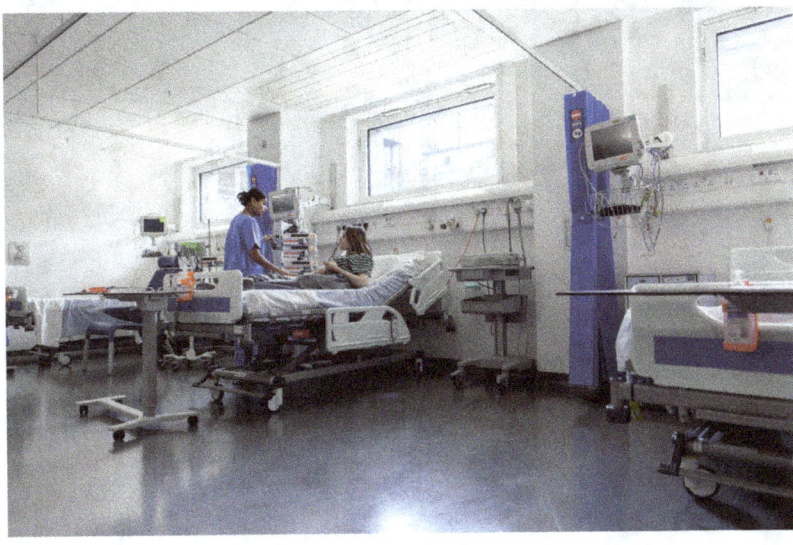

A hospital

Social care settings

Setting	What it does
Community centre	Local centre which focuses on the well-being of the local community. They provide activities to help people stay connected and gain new skills. They also offer classes, informal support and advice.
Day centre	Centres which provide support and activities to vulnerable people during the day. This benefits the service user but helps support informal carers by providing respite care. They can provide support for older people, people with disabilities, people with learning disabilities and people with mental health needs.
Food bank	Provide food and other basic supplies to people who are struggling financially to buy their own. Rely heavily on charitable donations.
Homeless shelter	Provide both temporary accommodation and other support for homeless people. This includes washing facilities, meals, and mental health and addiction support.
Residential care home	Provides long-term care to people who are no longer able to live in their own homes even with support. They provide support with washing, dressing, meals, activities and social activities. Residential homes do not usually have nurses on their staff.
Retirement home	Supported home for people, usually over the age of 55. They provide a safe environment, communal areas, emergency call systems and activities. Social care support provided by care assistants can be available but is not the main purpose of the retirement home.
Social services department	Department run by the local authority which assesses needs and arranges appropriate support for vulnerable people, including children and their families, and vulnerable adults. One of their most important roles is in safeguarding.
Support group	Groups of people that are struggling with similar issues. They are often run by people with the same challenge. Groups could include those for people with mental health issues, informal carers, bereaved individuals and people recovering from an addiction.

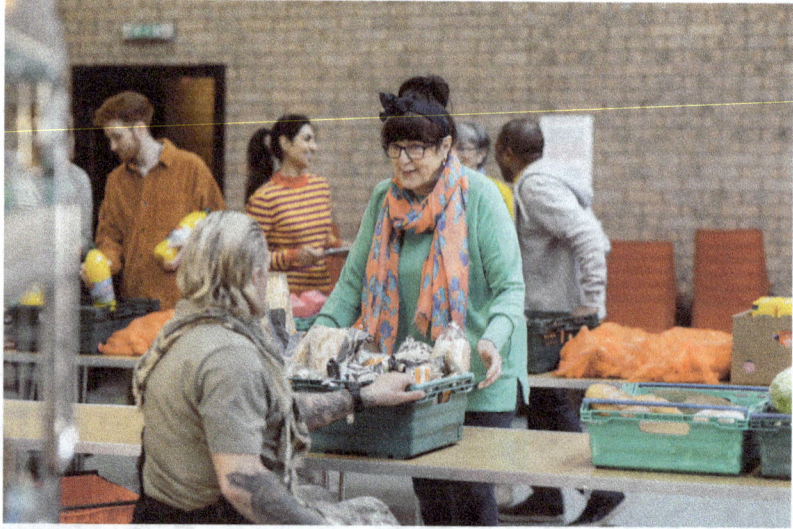

A food bank

1: Equality, diversity, and rights in health and social care settings

1.1 Diversity

Diversity refers to the differences between people in society. There are many aspects of diversity that you need to know about. You also need to know how each of the different groups can be supported in health and social care settings.

Age

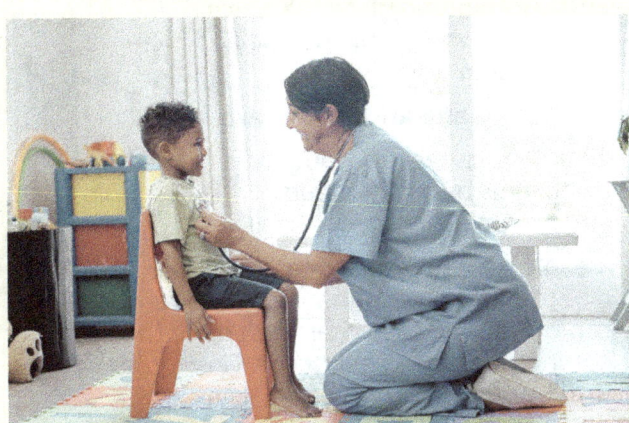

Overview

- Support is needed for children because they are still developing physically and emotionally.
- Older adults can often have long-term health conditions which affect their health and their ability to look after themselves.
- Both groups can be vulnerable and may require safeguarding.

Support in health and social care

- Support for children includes paediatric health services, CAMHS to support mental health, residential homes and foster care may also be needed.
- Children and their families are supported by children's social care services.
- All services that support children are responsible for safeguarding.
- Adult health is supported by GP services; they may need treatment and care in a hospital.
- Adult social care is supported by adult social services.

Cultural differences

Overview

- People from the same culture can share the same religion, language, customs, values, traditions and ways of behaving.
- A person's culture influences how they see themselves.
- If health and social care services do not take account of a person's culture, the individual will feel excluded.

Support in health and social care

- Personalised care plans, created with the service user, are more likely to respect their cultural needs.
- Where an individual has a different language, an interpreter or translation services may be necessary.
- Staff in all health and social care services should be given cultural awareness training so that they do not unintentionally discriminate against someone.

Disability

Overview

- An individual has a disability if they have difficulty carrying out daily activities because of a physical, mental, sensory or cognitive impairment.
- Environments and services that are not designed well make it harder for the individual to carry out day-to-day tasks.
- Services that take account of disabilities, and put things in place to reduce the difficulties, will enable people and increase their trust in the service.

Support in health and social care

- Buildings can take account of physical disabilities by having ramps, wide corridors and automatic doors.
- People who struggle to communicate due to sensory or cognitive impairment can be supported by staff who tailor their communication to suit needs. This could include short sentences and visual aids.
- Services may need specialist equipment such as hoists and mobility aids for physically disabled people.
- Alternative formats can be made available by settings for the information they provide, such as large print, braille and audio versions.
- Activities provided should be adapted to meet different needs.

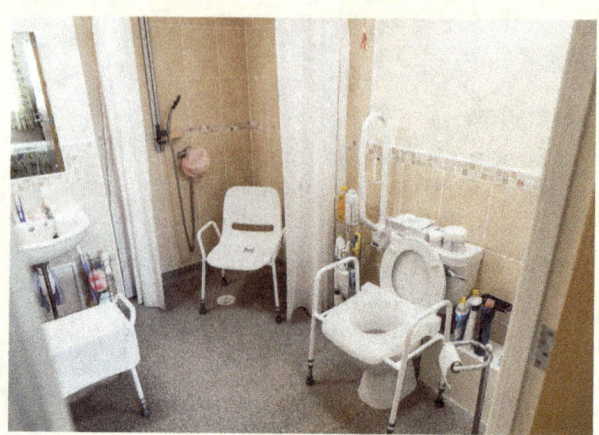

Bathroom adapted for a physically disabled person

Dress

Overview

- People wear clothes that reflect their culture, religion and personal beliefs as well as their personal choice.
- The hijab (headscarf) or the niqab (face veil) can be worn by Muslim women to show modesty.
- The thobe (long robe) can be worn by Muslim men to represent purity and modesty. It is often white.
- The sari (long cloth wrapped around the body, pictured) is worn by Hindu women.
- The dhoti (garment that wraps around the waist and legs) is a traditional garment worn by Hindu men.
- A turban is worn by Sikh men and symbolises religious devotion.
- A kippah is a small cap worn by Jewish men, especially when in a synagogue or during prayer and other religious events.
- A tallit is a Jewish prayer shawl worn around the shoulders during worship.
- A kimono is a traditional Japanese robe worn by both men and women.
- An abaya is a long, flowing cloak worn by women from some Middle Eastern countries as a sign of modesty.

Support in health and social care

- Religious and cultural dress should be respected in the uniform policies for health and social care workers.
- Health and social care settings should accept clothing choices and celebrate and educate service users and staff on the differences.
- Clothing provided by settings should be appropriate for people's age, cultural identity and physical needs.

Ethnicity

Overview

- A person's ethnicity relates to a shared background. This can include language, traditions, ancestry, religion and cultural identity.
- However, people from the same ethnic group can also have different cultures and religions.
- Some health conditions can be more *prevalent* in specific ethnic groups due to genetic or lifestyle factors.

Support in health and social care

- People who work in health and social care settings should not make assumptions about health needs or culture based on ethnicity.
- However, medical professionals need to be aware of the health patterns of different ethnic groups to ensure accurate diagnosis and the best treatments, e.g. prevalence of sickle cell disease for people with African or Caribbean heritage.
- Social care services need to ensure that ethnicity and culture are taken into account, such as for traditional diets.

Education

Overview

- Service users will have a variety of different educational backgrounds.
- Older people may have left school at a younger age (before 1944, school leaving age was 14, after 2023 it was 18).
- A person's education influences *health outcomes* greatly as it can affect their understanding of health advice.

Support in health and social care

- Services need to make information accessible to people from all educational backgrounds, such as having simpler information for people with poor literacy levels.
- Visual aids may help some groups of people.
- Health promotion should be tailored to someone's educational background and presented in a way that will be understood and accepted.

Family structure

Overview

- A nuclear family consists of two parents and children.
- Cohabiting families are where parents live together but are not married.
- Single-parent families are where one parent raises the child/children.
- Blended families are when children from previous relationships are part of the new family.
- Adoptive families are when children are adopted and brought up by non-biological parents.
- Same-sex families have parents of the same gender.
- Foster families are where children are fostered either short or long-term.
- Multigenerational families are where different generations of the family live in the same house.

Support in health and social care

- Health and social care services must avoid assumptions about a person's family structure.
- They should use inclusive language to build trust.
- Care plans should involve relevant family members regardless of the family structure – those people important to the individual.

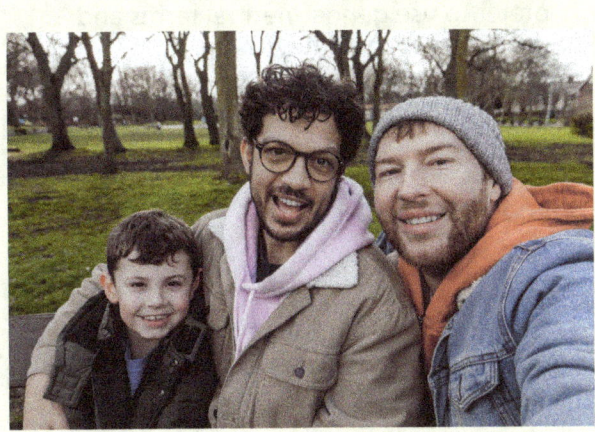

Food and special dietary requirements

Overview

- Some religious groups have dietary laws and preferences, such as halal (Muslim), kosher (Jewish), vegetarianism (Hindu), or fasting.
- Vegetarian and vegan diets need to pay attention to protein content to avoid adverse health implications.
- Some diets are required for specific medical needs, such as low carbohydrate for diabetes, low protein for kidney disease, low cholesterol for heart disease and low salt for high blood pressure. (Note: this is a greatly simplified overview!)
- The dietary needs of people change with age. Younger people need nutrients to grow, such as proteins and calcium, but older people also need plenty of protein to reduce muscle loss.
- Some people have food allergies or intolerances, such as reactions to glucose, gluten, nuts and shellfish.

Support in health and social care

- Health and social care services need to plan menus that take account of religious and cultural practices.
- Clear labelling is needed to avoid allergic reactions. People providing food need to be aware of people's allergies and intolerances to certain food so they are not given something by mistake that would be bad for them.
- Food should be appropriate for the age of the service user.
- Some individuals need personalised nutritional plans for their medical needs.

Gender/gender reassignment

Overview

- Gender refers to the roles, identities and behaviour that society associates with being male, female or non-binary.
- A person's gender is not always the same as their biological sex. A transgender person has a different gender identity to their biological sex.
- Gender reassignment is when a transgender person takes steps to transition to live as the gender they identify with.
- Gender and gender reassignment are protected characteristics under the Equality Act 2010.
- A non-binary person may not exclusively identify as either male or female and may prefer to use gender-neutral terms and pronouns such as they/them.

Support in health and social care

- Health and social care services should find out people's preferred pronouns and use them
- Gender-neutral facilities, such as unisex toilets and inclusive forms and questionnaires, should be provided.
- Staff should be trained on how to support people in a way that supports their gender identity and reduces discrimination.
- Preferences around gender should be protected – for example, some women may prefer female carers.

Language

Overview

- Many different languages are spoken in the UK.
- Relying just on English reduces accessibility to health and social care services.
- If there are language barriers, individuals may not understand care and treatment options open to them or may not be able to follow medical advice accurately.

Support in health and social care

- Information should be provided in different languages.
- Interpreters and translators should be available if possible.
- In areas where a particular language is more common, health and social care services should also employ staff that speak that language.
- Staff should be trained in how to communicate in a way that improves understanding for people who do not speak English well, such as avoiding jargon.

Music

Overview
- Music improves mental wellbeing.
- Music preferences can reflect a person's cultural, religious or personal identity.
- Playing familiar or traditional music can bring back memories and help reduce stress as well as promoting inclusion.

Support in health and social care
- Health and social care services should take account of their service users' preferences and diversity when they choose music to play.
- Music therapy sessions can be tailored to people's individual needs.
- Personal playlists can be created to reflect an individual's preferences – help can be obtained from family if the individual has dementia.

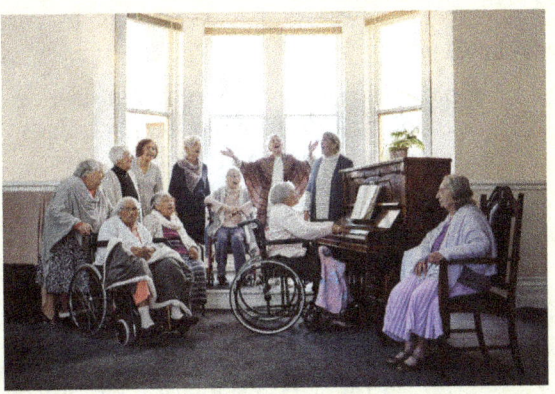

Residents of a home enjoying music together

- Activities could include cultural and religious music to help encourage people to learn and embrace other cultures and promote inclusivity.

Race

Overview
- Race is a social construct, which has been applied to people by society based on perceived physical characteristics.
- Race is different to ethnicity.
- Racial groups include white, black and Asian.
- Racial groups include individuals from many different ethnic and cultural backgrounds.

Support in health and social care
- Health and social care services should be aware of different health patterns to ensure appropriate diagnosis and treatment.
- They should employ a diverse workforce to represent the needs of all their service users.
- Care environments should reflect diverse backgrounds.

Example of race	Example of ethnicity
White	Roma
Asian	Punjabi
Black	British-Jamaican

Sexuality and sexual orientation

Overview
- Sexuality is about a person's sexual feelings, and includes sexual orientation.
- Sexual orientation is who someone is sexually or romantically attracted to. Some commonly recognised sexual orientations include:
  - » Heterosexual – attracted to the opposite gender.
  - » Homosexual – attracted to the same gender.
  - » Bisexual – attracted to more than one gender.
  - » Asexual – have limited sexual attraction but can have romantic feelings and relationships.
- The term LGBTQ+ refers to lesbian, gay, bisexual, transgender, queer/questioning. The 'plus' is inclusive of all other identities.

Support in health and social care
- Staff should be trained in all aspects related to equality to reduce prejudice and discrimination.
- Services should respect confidentiality around sexual orientation.
- Language used should be inclusive to help all individuals feel accepted.
- It is important to avoid assuming that someone is heterosexual and treating them as if they were unless you are told otherwise.
- Settings should create a welcoming environment such as through the use of rainbow flags and inclusive materials.

Religion or belief

Overview

- Religion and belief can greatly influence a person's daily life, values, food choices, routines and even healthcare choices.
- The largest religions include Christianity, Islam, Judaism, Hinduism, Buddhism and Sikhism.
- Some people have non-religious beliefs and may be atheist or agnostics.
- Religious practices can include worship, prayer, fasting, festivals and dietary restrictions.

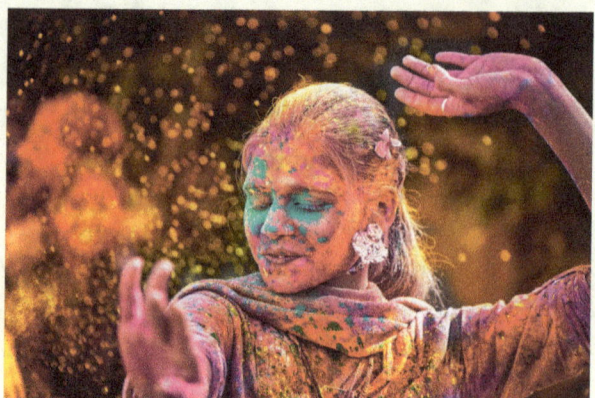

Woman taking part in the Hindu festival of Holi

Support in health and social care

- Care plans should take account of religious practices such as prayer times, dietary needs and important festivals.
- Many health and social care settings have multi-faith rooms for prayer and invite religious leaders to support their service users.
- Staff should be trained to understand key customs and beliefs across the different religions.

Socioeconomic background

Overview

- Socioeconomic background includes income, education, occupation and social class.
- People from lower socioeconomic backgrounds are statistically more likely to have poorer health outcomes and a shorter life expectancy.
- This could be due to reduced access to healthcare, lack of access to nutritious food, poorer housing and less knowledge about healthy lifestyles.

Support in health and social care

- Health and social care services should offer flexible appointment times to accommodate shift workers and busy schedules
- The NHS provides free healthcare at the point of service to overcome some socioeconomic barriers.
- Schemes such as the prescription exemption certificate and voucher systems for eye care help make prescriptions and eye care more affordable.
- Services like food banks, homeless shelters and benefit advice centres aim to support people on low incomes.
- Services should offer clear information about what people are entitled to so that they do not miss out.

1.2 Equality

Equality
- Individuals must be given the same opportunities regardless of differences.
- They must be treated fairly and with respect.
- They must be treated according to their beliefs.

Being given the same opportunity is not the same as being treated equally – it is where barriers are removed or reduced, so the individual can still achieve the same as others.

- **Importance of equality** – improves people's emotional wellbeing, provides extra support where needed to gain the same opportunities as others. Under the Equality Act 2010 it is a legal requirement that services promote equality.
- **Negative impact of not applying equality** – health and social care needs may not be met, some groups will have poorer health outcomes than others, some groups may even die younger. Settings that do not promote equality may be prosecuted and will get a bad reputation.
- **Link between equality and diversity** – a diverse society includes people from different backgrounds with different beliefs and preferences. Equality means ensuring everyone, regardless of their differences, gets the same chances in life and health and wellbeing as others.

How settings promote equality

- Accessible layouts to suit different physical needs e.g. ramps and lifts.
- Hearing loops to support people with hearing aids.
- Translation services to support people with different languages.
- Employing staff who can speak different languages.
- Training for staff in equality and diversity.
- Food choices that take account of different religious and cultural needs, personal preferences and medical needs.
- Provide advocates so that people who do not feel able to speak up for themselves can still have their voices heard.

1.3 Rights

Rights are protected by law and are written into the codes of practice that health and social care professionals work by. These rights are set out in the table below:

Right	Summary
Choice	Service users should be able to make their own decisions about how they live their lives, what they would like to eat and wear, where they want to live, and what type of medical treatment to have.
Confidentiality	Personal information kept by health and social care settings must be protected so that only people that need the information to provide care can access it. Consent must be gained from the service user before it is shared.
Consultation	People should be asked their opinions when decisions are being made about them. They should be fully informed of all the facts and possible consequences of the decisions so they can make an informed decision.
Equal and fair treatment	All service users should be able to expect to receive the same high-quality care and support as everyone else regardless of their background, beliefs and preferences.
Protection from abuse and harm	All service users should be protected from abuse, neglect and harm, such as during an accident.

How rights are promoted in health and social care

- Providing person-centred care is where a care plan is drawn up with full involvement of the individual and takes into account their differences, religious beliefs and preferences.
- **Communication** must be good and be adapted to the service user's needs where necessary.
- Service users must always be given a **choice**, such as what time to get up, or what to eat for lunch.
- Staff should be trained so that they can **promote the rights** of people in their care.
- Service users must be **consulted** on all important decisions. Extra time and support may be needed to do this with people who struggle to understand.
- Provide or encourage **advocates** to promote the rights of individuals.
- Health and social care workers should **follow legislation**, including the Health and Care Act 2022, to safeguard service users.

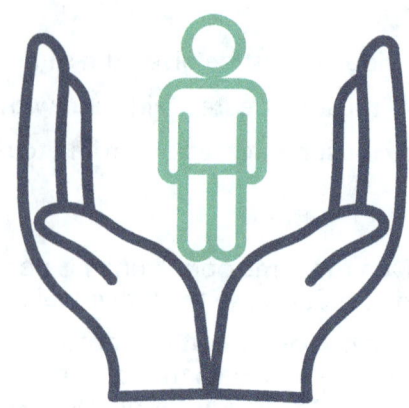

Person centred care

1.4 Discrimination in health and social care environments

Prejudice is when someone has an opinion or makes a judgement about someone without having the knowledge or experience to be able to form the opinion or make the judgement.

» For example, deciding what people can do, or what they would want to do, without having met them and instead basing it on some characteristic such as race or gender.

When someone treats someone unfavourably because of their prejudice, they **discriminate** against them. The two main types of discrimination are:

- **Direct discrimination** – when someone actively treats a person less favourably because of a characteristic they have.
- **Indirect discrimination** – when a policy, procedure, rule or way of working applies to everyone but accidentally has a more negative impact for a specific group of people. For example, a work dress code that bans wearing anything on the head would prevent some people from following their faith.
- **Intentional discrimination** – when the person who is discriminating against someone knows that they are treating someone less favourably.
- **Unintentional discrimination** – when the person or organisation that is discriminating is unaware that their actions or rules are having a negative impact on particular groups of people because of a characteristic they have.

Direct discrimination		Indirect discrimination	
Treating someone less favourably because of a characteristic they have		Where a policy negatively impacts some groups more than others. (Note: most indirect discrimination is unintentional)	
Intentional	**Unintentional**	**Intentional**	**Unintentional**
e.g. refusing to provide care for a service user because they belong to a particular ethnic group.	e.g. assuming a wheelchair user cannot take part in an activity so not offering them the opportunity.	e.g. setting promotion eligibility rules knowing that they exclude groups that cannot work full-time such as carers or parents.	e.g. a GP surgery introducing an online only booking system without understanding that it excludes several groups.

A basis of discrimination is the reason or characteristic that leads to people treating them less favourably. The main bases of discrimination are shown in the table below:

Basis	Outline
Race	People make assumptions about people based on their race or ethnicity. These assumptions lead to unfair treatment. Example: Black British women are less likely to be offered epidurals during birth.
Age	Younger adults or teenagers and older adults are the most likely people to be discriminated against because of their age. This happens when people base their expectations on stereotypes of people in the same age group. Examples: » The concerns of young people dismissed as being overdramatic. » Older people not being offered the same diagnostic tests as a younger adult and their symptoms are dismissed as "old age".
Culture and religion	Stereotypical views of people from different cultures can lead to unequal treatment. Lack of cultural awareness may cause insult or make it harder for a person to follow their culture. Example: » Health and social care settings may not provide choices that meet a person's cultural needs.
Disability	People make assumptions about people's abilities or lack of them when they know someone is disabled. People may also assume that if they cannot see a disability, it is not there – these are known as **invisible disabilities**. People may not take a person's disability into consideration when planning services. Examples: » Refusing to provide a service to disabled people because it would mean that the service would have to make reasonable adjustments.
Gender	People have stereotypes about gender roles. Medical research has sometimes been conducted on men and does not match the needs of women. Gender-specific needs are sometimes missed. Example: » Women in a family are presumed to be happy with the caring role, leading to less respite support being offered.
Socio-economic background	People in low socioeconomic groups often have overlooked disadvantages that affect their health. They also have limited access to services due to cost barriers (despite the NHS). Example: » Appointments during work hours exclude people who are less able to take time off work.
Sexual orientation	Non-heterosexual people are more likely to be discriminated against because of their sexuality. This can be direct or indirect, if it is assumed people are heterosexual, leading to people feeling misunderstood. Example: » Assuming two people of the same gender are friends rather than partners can lead to a lack of the same visiting rights as other couples.

The way people discriminate against people is called discriminatory behaviour. Here are some examples:

- **Abuse** is when people are deliberately treated badly. Different forms of abuse:
    - **Verbal** – using words to upset or control someone else.
    - **Physical** – deliberately harming someone physically, including hitting, punching, kicking and burning.
    - **Mental** or **psychological** – threatening or making someone feel unworthy or useless.
    - **Neglect** – where a person's needs are ignored, including not providing them with food, drink, medication, protection or social stimulation.
    - **Financial** – misusing someone's money or property, including theft.
- **Being patronised** is acting superior to someone or treating them like they do not have the abilities they do. It includes talking down to someone or making decisions on their behalf without their input.

- **Breach of health and safety** is where a person's safety needs are ignored, leading to harm to the individual.
- **Bullying** is when someone is repeatedly treated badly. It includes humiliating, hurting or intimidating them.
- **Inadequate care** is when people from a particular group are not given care that meets their needs. This leads to poorer health outcomes and low self-esteem.
- **Stereotyping** or **labelling** is where people decide that because an individual has a certain characteristic, other characteristics, behaviours or beliefs also apply to the individual.

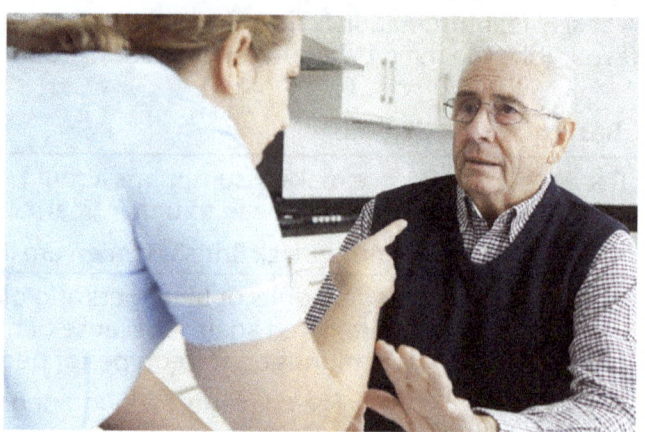

Service user being bullied by carer

1.5 Potential impacts on individuals of discrimination

Discrimination has many different impacts on the people who are being discriminated against. These impacts can be physical, intellectual, emotional, social or financial (PIESF):

- **Physical impacts** lead to harm to an individual or a deterioration in their condition.
- **Intellectual impacts** affect an individual's ability to learn, process information or develop skills. It affects their cognitive abilities and development.
- **Emotional impacts** damage a person's self-esteem, mental health or emotional wellbeing.
- **Social impacts** affect people's ability to have or maintain relationships with other people or take part in community life or activity. It affects their social belonging.
- **Financial impacts** – leads to loss of money or property, leading to economic disadvantage for that individual.

Physical	Intellectual	Emotional	Social	Financial
Harm or poor health due to poor treatment	Limitations on learning, development of skills or cognitive processing	Damage to self-esteem, confidence or emotional well-being	Restriction of social interaction or involvement in community due to discrimination	Causing economic disadvantage due to procedures
e.g. poor health due to dietary needs being ignored	e.g. being excluded from an activity due to learning disabilities	e.g. an older person begin patronised	e.g. LGBTQ+ groups not being excluded from planning outings at a care home	e.g. discrimination leading to job loss

Some specific impacts of discrimination

Impact	Details
Disempowerment	Where the individual no longer has control over decisions about their life. • Physical – lack of involvement from individuals can lead to poor treatment decisions. • Intellectual – individual no longer using cognitive abilities to make decisions. • Emotional – may feel worthless as their opinion is not sought. • Social – may withdraw from social activities or relationships. • Financial – may not feel able to ask for financial support.
Fear	When someone is being mistreated, they fear the consequences because they suspect the discrimination will lead to harm and that complaining might make the situation worse. • Emotional – fear will cause constant anxiety, which will affect emotional wellbeing and cause stress. • Social – fear of being mistreated can cause people to withdraw from relationships.
Illness	If discrimination has prevented a person from receiving the right treatment, they may become ill, or their illness may become worse. Anxiety may also cause illness. • Physical – untreated conditions will cause physical condition to deteriorate. • Emotional – deteriorating health and illness can lead to depression. • Social – can cause isolation and loneliness if people lose independence and are unable to do things they used to enjoy. • Financial – the individual may not be able to work due to the illness and may need to pay for medications or care.
Injury	Not taking account of someone's needs or treating them roughly due to discrimination can cause physical injury. • Physical – injury is physical harm.
Low self-confidence	Where an individual no longer believes in their own judgement and abilities. • Intellectual – lack of confidence in their abilities leads to them avoiding mentally challenging tasks due to fear of failure. • Emotional – feelings of doubt will lead to anxiety and possibly depression. • Social – they may worry about what other people think of them and avoid social contact for fear of being judged.
Low self-esteem	Where someone has a lack of self-worth and self-respect. • Intellectual – less likely to be curious about things or try new things. • Emotional – leads to sadness and hopelessness; they also feel less deserving. • Social – may withdraw from social activities due to feeling bad about themselves or feelings of shame.
Physical harm	Includes direct injury due to the discrimination or neglect of their needs leading to health consequences. • Physical – can include bruising, infections, malnutrition and poor skin conditions due to poor care.

Impact	Details
Poor physical health	Physical health may deteriorate due to neglect of physical and health needs, or anxiety and stress may impact on physical health. • Physical – can lead to chronic conditions, a deterioration of existing health conditions and malnutrition. • Intellectual – inability to concentrate and poor motivation. • Emotional – anxiety and depression. • Social – may be less able to participate in social activities due to physical harm. • Financial – may not be able to work, may have extra health and social care related costs.
Poor mental health	Can lead to long-term psychological harm. • Physical – poor mental health can lead to self-neglect and self-harming, which impacts physical health. • Intellectual – it will be harder to engage in intellectual activities. • Emotional – can lead to depression, anxiety, PTSD and suicidal thoughts. • Social – may withdraw socially. • Financial – may not be able to work due to mental health problems.
Unfair treatment	Where an individual receives lower quality care or support than others. • Physical – leads to poor health. • Intellectual – may not be given the opportunity to make decisions about their care. • Emotional – leads to feelings of rejection and distress. • Social – may become isolated.

Study Tips!

- Understanding the roles of each health and social care setting will help you understand how they work to support diversity in their setting.
- You will need to know how each of the aspects of diversity can be supported within health and social care settings.
- Remember that some health and social care settings are aimed at specific age groups, such as residential homes for older people, whereas others will need to support people from all age groups, such as a GP surgery.
- Remember that not all people with a disability have a physical disability, so some adjustments to settings or services will take account of non-physical disabilities.
- Culture, ethnicity and race are connected to each other but are different. Culture relates to shared values and beliefs; ethnicity is about sharing a common background, while race is how people are categorised by society into groups based on physical features.
- It is very important to remember that promoting equality is not the same as treating everybody the same. Health and social care services need to put in more support to some people based on their needs. Treating people the same would mean that some people would not have their needs met.
- You may need to be able to read a scenario and pick out which rights are or are not being supported within the scenario.
- Direct discrimination can be intentional or unintentional. Indirect discrimination can be intentional but is more likely to be unintentional. In health and social care settings, unintentional indirect discrimination is likely if settings have not carefully reviewed their policies to make sure they are not accidentally discriminating.
- When thinking about the impacts of discrimination it is often easier to think about physical and emotional impacts. Remember to use PIESF to also think of intellectual, social and financial impacts.

Important terms!

Primary care – Healthcare that is the first point of contact for a member of the community. Examples include GP surgeries, community nurses and community midwives. A hospital is an example of secondary healthcare.

Secondary care – Specialist services which patients need to be referred to.

Service user – An individual who uses health and social care services.

Respite care – Short-term care to give informal/family carers a break from their caring duties. It might mean that an individual spends one week every few weeks in a care home or hospice to be looked after while their unpaid carers get a break.

Local authority – A government organisation that is responsible for the public services for a particular geographical area of the UK. They run services like waste collection, education and social services within the area.

Safeguarding – Procedures and activities to protect the safety and well-being of vulnerable people. It aims to prevent harm (such as abuse) and to deal appropriately with suspicions of abuse to prevent further harm.

Informal carer – Someone who supports an individual who is unable to fully care for themselves but does not get paid for this work. It is usually a family member, friend or neighbour.

Paediatric – Healthcare that relates to children from birth up to the age of 18.

CAMHS – Child and Adolescent Mental Health Services are mental health services for children and young people run by the NHS.

Cognitive – The mental processes that are involved in understanding things. It can include thinking, remembering, problem solving and judging.

Prevalent – A word used to describe how widespread a particular disease is at a particular time. It includes how many people currently have the disease. If a disease is prevalent, it means that a lot of people currently have the disease.

Health outcomes – A change in health status following healthcare interventions. A good health outcome would be complete recovery.

Halal – Comes from the Arabic word for 'permissible' and refers to food, practices and products that comply with Islamic law. Halal meat must be killed in a specific way.

Kosher – Comes from the Hebrew word for 'fit' and refers to food that complies with Jewish dietary laws.

Inclusion – Where everybody is included in an activity or service regardless of any differences they may have from others in the group. It includes encouraging and enabling people to participate.

Atheist – A person who does not believe in any god.

Agnostic – A person who feels that it is not possible to know whether there is a god or not.

Prescription exemption certificate – A certificate that allows certain individuals to have free prescriptions. People may get one due to having specific medical conditions or being on a low income.

Hearing loop – Also known as an induction system. It is installed in public places including communal areas of health and social care settings. It helps make speech easier to hear for people wearing hearing aids. They need to turn their hearing aid to the 'T' setting for it to work.

Advocate – Someone who speaks up on behalf of a vulnerable person; this means that person's views are heard and considered.

Code of practice – A set of guidelines or standards expected of a particular profession such as nursing.

Informed decision – Understanding all the factors that affect a decision, including possible consequences of a particular choice. It will include knowing the benefits and risks of the decision.

Person-centred care – A way of providing care that respects an individual's differences, preferences, needs and values.

Reasonable adjustment – Changes made to a setting, service or someone's employment to overcome barriers due to disabilities.

PTSD – Post-Traumatic Stress Disorder is a mental health condition brought about by experiencing a traumatic event. Symptoms include anxiety, nightmares and flashbacks to the event. It can also be triggered by witnessing a traumatic event, even if the person was not directly involved in it.

Recap Questions

1. Describe the diversity of religion and beliefs. How might this be supported in a health and social care setting?
2. What is equality?
3. Explain what is meant by confidentiality.
4. Why is the right to consultation important in a health and social care setting?
5. Explain the difference between prejudice and discrimination.
6. Give an example of gender discrimination in a health and social care setting.
7. Describe the difference between intentional and unintentional discrimination.
8. Give an example of unintentional discrimination that could occur in a GP surgery.
9. Give two examples of a social care setting.
10. What does gender reassignment refer to?
11. What impact can socioeconomic background have on health outcomes?
12. Why is being patronising an example of discriminatory behaviour?
13. Give an example of psychological abuse.
14. Give an example of a health and social care setting where financial abuse could occur.
15. Give an example of a type of discrimination that can lead to poor mental health.
16. What are the emotional impacts of fear?
17. What does ethnicity mean?
18. What does atheist mean? How could this be supported in a setting?

Revision Quiz

1. Who in a residential children's home might need an enhanced DBS check?
2. How can a health care professional demonstrate commitment?
3. Why is compassion important for a GP?
4. How can someone with a visual impairment be supported in a social care setting?
5. Give two types of health and safety training might care home staff need?
6. What are the nine protected characteristics under the Equality Act?
7. Why do people in care homes need to be trained to use hoists?
8. The Children's Act gives children a right to an advocate. Explain what this means.
9. Why should cleaning materials be locked away in a residential care home?
10. What must be reported to the UKHSA?
11. Why does a hospital need a Data Protection Officer?
12. What impact does the Health and Safety at Work Act have on residents of a care home?

Assessment practice

1. Give two ways that health and social care services can support people from different cultures. (2)
2. Describe one way of supporting people with cognitive disabilities in health and social care settings. (2)
3. Explain why music choices based on a person's culture can help support them in a health and social care setting. (2)
4. Explain why hiring workers from different races will improve equality and diversity in the setting. (2)
5. Give three ways health and social care services can promote equality (3).
6. Choose two correct ways to provide health and social care users with choice. (2)

    A Give clear information about the decision being made.

    B Ensure that the service user is making the right decision by letting them know if they seem to be choosing the wrong option.

    C Offer a single option to make it easier for people with cognitive difficulties to decide.

    D Respect the person's choice even if you do not agree with them.

    E Always provide information in writing for everyone.

7. Give two reasons why maintaining confidentiality is important in health and social care. (2)
8. State two reasons why health and social care professionals should listen to the views of an individual before making important decisions about them. (2)
9. Describe what equal and fair treatment is. (3)
10. Choose the two most appropriate ways to provide care to people of different age groups: (2)

    A Give a younger person time before allocating resources as their symptoms may go away on their own.

    B When communicating with older people, use short and simple sentences so they can understand more easily.

    C Base treatments and care on the individual's needs rather than their age.

    D Provide choices of activity for a younger service user based on what you know younger people like.

    E Allocate time and resources based on the person's individual needs.

11. Explain why setting up mobile health screening units in some parts of a city can affect early diagnosis of serious conditions in people of a low socioeconomic group. (3)
12. Describe how considering different educational levels of people in different socio-economic groups when giving health advice can affect health outcomes. (2)
13. Describe what neglect is. (2)
14. Give two ways in which discrimination can lead to harm in health and social care settings. (2)
15. State one financial impact of disempowerment. (1)
16. Give two reasons why discrimination may lead to injury. (2)
17. Give three reasons why discrimination can lead to poor physical health. (3)
18. Explain how unfair treatment as a result of discrimination can lead to financial impacts. (3)

A community centre is keen to promote equality to meet the needs of the diverse local population. It has disabled access and a translation service. The staff are trained in health and safety. Notices and leaflets are written in different languages, braille, large print and easy read. There is a canteen which provides a range of sandwiches, salads and chips as well as various drinks and desserts. One user of the service is 62-year-old Ralph, who is deaf, has coeliac disease and struggles to make connections with others.

19. a) Discuss how well the community centre is promoting equality (6)

   b) Explain how treating people according to their needs will help support Ralph. (4)

Sarah is of Indian descent and is Hindu. She is 72 years old and has just moved into Hill View residential home due to her severe arthritis which has affected her mobility. One member of staff is very rough when helping her to get out of bed, so she now has bruises on her arms. Some staff promote dietary choices that meet her cultural needs but some do not, so she often has to settle for an omelette as the vegetarian option. Some have ignored her requests for a better choice while others have openly mocked her. She has noticed that Rachel, who is from a lower socioeconomic background usually has to wait until last for assistance. Edith, the eldest resident, is often treated as if she has dementia even though she does not. Sarah was pleased to see that different cultural festivals are celebrated at the home. She has enjoyed learning about other cultures. The staff have told her that the home is going to put on equality and diversity training.

20. a) Explain how different types of discriminatory behaviour occurs in the home. (4)

   b) Justify why equality and diversity training is essential in preventing discrimination. (4)

   c) Discuss the extent to which the home is managing to prevent discrimination. Consider both successful ways of working and where discrimination is still taking place. (9)

2: Managing hazards, health and safety in health and social care settings

2.1 Potential hazards in health and social care settings

- **Hazards** are things that could cause someone harm if the circumstances are right.
- A **risk** is the chance that the hazard will cause harm.

You need to know the following hazards in health and social care settings, which settings they are most likely to relate to and who might be affected by each.

Biological hazards come from living organisms and include **body fluids** and **diseases** or **infections**.

Hazard	Examples	Who is most at risk?
Bodily fluids	Urine Faeces Blood Saliva Vomit Clinical waste	People who work in health and social care settings as they will need to work with these hazards. All service users who may become exposed by accident due to poor health and safety procedures.
Diseases/infections	Infections caused by bacteria, viruses, fungi and protozoa, such as: • Flu • Covid-19 • MRSA • Norovirus • Head lice and scabies	Health and social care workers. Service users who are more vulnerable due to being young or very old or due to having a weaker immune system such as people with HIV.

Chemical hazards are chemicals that could be ingested, inhaled or exposed to people's skin causing serious health problems. They include **medicines** and **cleaning materials**.

Hazard	Details and examples	Who is most at risk?
Medicines	Tablets, liquid medication, skin patches. Medication can be given in the wrong dose or taken by people they are not prescribed for.	Service users who are confused and may take the wrong medication. Service users who are given the wrong medication by accident. Health and social care workers with inadequate training.
Cleaning materials	Can be dangerous if mixed as they might give off poisonous gases. Could be ingested by vulnerable service users. Can cause harm with exposure to skin, eyes, mouth and nose.	People with dementia may accidentally drink cleaning chemicals. Service users may be at risk if cleaning chemicals are not stored properly. Domestic staff if they have not been trained or do not have the appropriate PPE.

Environmental hazards are due to factors that surround the setting such as the conditions inside or outside the building. They include **temperature** and **noise**.

Hazard	Examples	Who is most at risk?
Temperature	Too hot – can cause heat exhaustion, heat stroke and dehydration. Too cold – can cause hypothermia.	Service users who cannot control their home's heating controls. Service users who are not mobile so cannot access drinks when needed. Workers who need to work in hot conditions for the sake of the service users and may not have time to drink enough fluids.
Noise	Can be disturbing and cause upset and mental health conditions. Noise at night can disrupt sleep. Examples: heart monitors and other equipment, loud TVs, people talking loudly due to hearing impairments, repair work on health and social care setting buildings.	Service users with mental health problems. Service users who have difficulty sleeping.

Working conditions are the conditions workers work in and the consequences of these conditions on the service users. Working conditions can affect the safety of **moving and handling** and includes the **equipment** used in the health and social care settings.

Hazard	Examples	Who is most at risk?
Moving and handling	Moving and handling equipment can cause harm if not used correctly. Poor moving and handling techniques can cause harm. Harm is more likely if staff have not been trained properly or if they are overworked and rush the task.	Service users who are being moved by staff. Health and social care workers who have not been trained properly or who are doing a lot of moving and handling of patients without sufficient breaks between.
Equipment	Moving and handling equipment e.g.: • Hoists • Machines such as cleaning machines • X-rays and other scanning equipment • Hospital beds • Needles	Children who may play on equipment. Service users who are having the equipment used on them. Workers who are using the machines.

Physical hazards include **slips and trips** and **radiation** exposure.

Hazard	Examples	Who is most at risk?
Slips and trips	Slipping on wet floors Tripping over obstacles, frayed carpets and cables Falling due to poor balance	Service users who slip or trip. Health and social care workers may try to catch a service user as they fall and cause themselves damage in the process.
Radiation	From scanning machines such as X-rays and CT scans The radiation from radiotherapy which is used to shrink cancerous tumours.	Pregnant women and their unborn child are at risk from x-rays and should only have these scans if absolutely necessary. Health and social care workers who operate the scanning machines or who carry out radiotherapy.

Poor working practices are when there are inadequate procedures, the procedures are not being carried out or staff are overworked and rush to get all their work done. Inadequate training and lack of equipment also contributes towards poor working practices.

Hazard	Examples	Who is most at risk?
Long working hours and breaks	Long working hours and not enough breaks lead to exhaustion and poor concentration in workers. Accidents and mistakes are more likely to happen.	Service users who are being cared for by overworked staff. The staff themselves may have an accident, may be more prone to illness or may go off work with stress.
Supervision	Less qualified and experienced staff need to be supervised by more experienced managers or colleagues. If supervision is inadequate it might lead to: • Workers doing tasks incorrectly • Workers doing tasks they are not trained to do • Anxiety in the staff as they are not sure what they should do	Service users may be exposed to incorrect treatment by an unsupervised member of staff leading to harm. Staff may feel they are not being supported and may leave the profession leading to staff shortages.

Lack of security systems mean that unauthorised people may get into a health and social care setting and cause harm to service users. It could also mean that vulnerable service users may leave the setting and be at risk of harm outside. This may not be noticed for some time in a busy setting.

Hazard	Examples	Who is most at risk?
Door/window locks	Prevent intruders entering the building and should be checked regularly, especially at night. They also prevent vulnerable service users from leaving.	Service users may be at risk from intruders who may steal from them or may deliberately cause them harm. Vulnerable service users like dementia patients or children may be at risk if they can freely leave the building as they could cross busy roads, get lost or encounter other people who may cause them harm.
Alarm systems	Alarms can trigger if external doors are opened so that staff are aware if someone has entered or if someone leaves. They can then check the credentials of visitors or check that vulnerable service users have not managed to get out.	Children. Service users with dementia. Newborn babies could be taken from the crib if an alarm is not on the crib or on the maternity ward door.

2.2 Possible impacts of hazards on individuals receiving or providing care

Hazards that are not controlled lead to several impacts on both service users and health and social care workers. Some examples are below:

Illness

- Being given the wrong medication can cause serious illness.
- Ingestion of cleaning chemicals such as by a child or someone with dementia.
- Inadequate care can cause stress which can lead to illness.
- Inadequate hydration in hot weather can lead to dehydration and is a serious health risk.
- Poor temperature control can lead to hyperthermia or hypothermia.
- Drafts and poor ventilation can lead to an increased risk of respiratory illnesses.

Infection

- Inadequate infection control can cause diseases to be passed on from ill patients to both service users and staff. Service users with weak immune systems are most at risk.
- Poor waste disposal can increase risk of exposure to infectious diseases.
- Dirty surfaces, due to inadequate cleaning, can increase the risk of cross contamination.
- Poor hygiene and lack of the correct PPE can infect staff and make them carriers for infections even if they do not get sick themselves.
- MRSA is a particular problem in health and social care settings and is spread when hygiene in the setting is poor.

Physical harm

- Slips and trips can lead to broken bones which can be especially serious in older people.
- Poor security can increase the risk of attacks to service users and staff.
- Cuts, grazes and bruises are more likely to both service users and staff if the staff are rushing.
- Incorrect use of machines, such as hoists, can lead to serious injuries such as crushing injuries.

Poor physical health

- Inadequate care can lead to poor hygiene, skin problems and weight changes in service users.
- Not positioning immobile service users correctly can lead to pressure ulcers which can cause serious harm and take a long time to heal.
- Incorrect manual handling techniques used over long periods of time can damage the body and lead to injuries and long-term sickness for staff.
- High workload can increase stress and weaken the immune system making illnesses and poor physical health more likely such as high blood pressure.

Poor mental health

- Unsafe environments lead to anxiety, depression and trauma.
- Poor health and safety can lead to mistrust of carers by the service users which may cause them to refuse care.
- Long working hours and regular exposure to traumatic events can lead to burnout in staff.
- Poor supervision can cause stress and mental health problems in staff.

Financial loss

- Service users and staff who are injured may no longer be able to work so suffer financial loss due to lower incomes.
- Service users who have been exposed to poor health and safety may feel they have no choice but to pay for private care which may use up all their savings.
- Injuries, illness, poor physical and mental health caused by inadequate health and safety may require regular medication which will cost money.
- People injured by hazards may need to pay carers to support them.
- Staff who are off work due to sickness following poor health and safety will be on a greatly reduced income.

Poor standard of care

- Inadequate health and safety may lead to staff going off sick or leaving. The resulting staff shortages may cause the remaining staff to rush and provide a poor standard of care.
- Rushed staff are more likely to miss signs of abuse, make errors in administering medication and working in other unsafe ways.
- Poor staffing levels leaves less time for training (CPD) so staff are less able to do things in the correct manner.

2.3 Health and safety management

Risk assessments are used to help manage risk.

» They are used to identify the hazards and risk of harm and to decide what measures should be taken to reduce the risk of harm.

Risk assessments reduce injury and harm in health and social care settings and are required by the law (see section 3).

Risk assessments identify some **control measures** that should be put in place to mitigate the risk.

Some examples include:

- **Infection control** which includes wearing PPE, good hygiene and thorough cleaning schedules
- Patient **safety protocols** may involve falls prevention strategies and protocols on how to handle medication safely
- **Fire safety** will include regular fire drills, robust evacuation plans and adequate extinguisher access and training
- **Manual handling safety** will rely on good training, appropriate equipment that is checked for safety before use and personalised care plans detailing how a specific service user should be moved.
- **Prevention of violence** will involve adequate security, training for staff and good visitor controls.

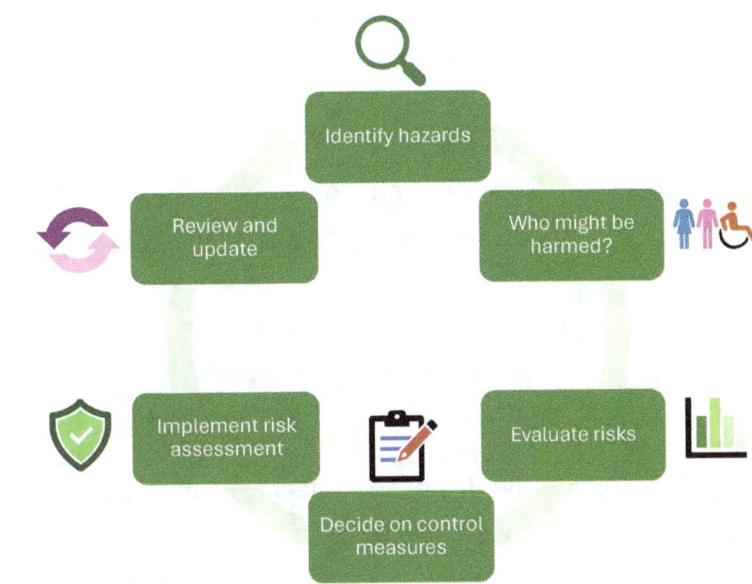

Methods health and social care settings use to minimise risk:

Method	Details	
Clear health and safety procedures	<ul><li>All settings must have health and safety policies and procedures.</li><li>They outline everybody's role in managing health and safety.</li><li>They state the training requirements of staff.</li></ul>	All workers know what they must do to reduce harm and accidents.
Keeping health and safety procedures up to date	<ul><li>Procedures should be reviewed to check they are still relevant and that they still comply with the latest legislation.</li><li>They should be reviewed at least annually.</li><li>Changes in legislation or incidents caused by poor health and safety should cause policies to be reviewed sooner.</li></ul>	The procedures and ways of working will comply with all legislation. Ways of working will keep up to date with latest best practice guidance. Policies and procedures can be updated to reflect learning from accidents that have happened at the setting.

Method	Details	
Staff training and supervision	Training should be made available and should be renewed regularly as set out in the health and safety procedures. Some health and safety training: • First aid • Fire safety • Manual handling • Health and hygiene • Infection control • Health and safety awareness • Administering of medication	Staff are regularly updates on the law and the latest best practice ways of working to reduce accidents and harm. Training reduces errors that lead to accidents. Protects both service users and staff. Increases confidence and competence of staff.
Displaying health and safety signs and information clearly	Information that must be displayed: • Health and safety legislation poster from the Health and Safety Executive (HSE). • Location of fire exits. • Hazard warning signs such as radiation warnings on x-ray room doors.	Reminds both service users and staff what is required by health and safety legislation. Gives details of whom to contact if there are concerns about health and safety. Enables everybody to find an exit in an emergency.
Dealing with hazards promptly	Examples include: • Cleaning up spills immediately before someone slips. • Removing broken equipment from use. • Reporting accidents and near misses. • Dealing with and reporting security breaches.	Prevents accidents. Required by health and safety law.
Use of Personal Protective Equipment	Examples of PPE include: • Disposable gloves • Plastic aprons • Face masks • Eye protection • Shoe covers • Overalls Not all PPE is needed for all tasks. PPE should be provided free by the employer.	Protects staff from infection and service users from cross contamination which prevents illness. Protects staff from other harmful substances such as chemicals.
Keeping areas cleaned and well maintained	• Regular cleaning schedules to maintain good hygiene standards. • Visual checks in relation to cleanliness. • Visual checks of equipment to check for faults before use. • Formal checks on equipment such as hoists (every 6 months) and portable electrical equipment (PAT testing) regularly depending on setting.	Reduces the spread of infection. Prevents use of broken equipment that could harm people. Testing electrical equipment can prevent fires and electric shocks.

2.4 Health and safety incidents in health and social care settings

Certain incidents are more likely to happen in health and social care settings. Putting plans in place in case these incidents occur and training staff on how to respond will ensure a much quicker and more effective response and can save lives.

Some possible incidents include:

- Accidents
- Emergences, including:
  - » Fire
  - » Flood
  - » Chemical or gas leak
  - » Outbreak of infectious diseases
  - » Missing persons

To deal with these incidents health and social care settings will need to:

- Have procedures in place for that incident so all staff know how to deal with it.
- Allocate staff to specific roles so that they can act quickly and automatically.
- Practice dealing with incidents such as by having fire drills.
- Having clear reporting and recording procedures so that the incident can be learned from.
- Follow-up and review incidents and procedures to further reduce risk in future.
- Report specific incidents to the relevant authorities including:
  - » Care Quality Commission (CQC)
  - » Health and Safety Executive (HSE)
  - » Emergency services including police, fire, ambulance
  - » Local authorities and their social service departments

Below is a table outlining the responses required for these incidents.

Incident	Response	Reporting requirements
Accidents	<ul><li>Call emergency services if required.</li><li>Carry out first aid.</li><li>Isolate the hazard (e.g. switch off electricity supply for an electrocution).</li><li>Clean up any spills to prevent further accidents.</li><li>Conduct an internal investigation later to see if policies need to be changed.</li></ul>	<ul><li>Record accident in the accident book (required by law)</li><li>Report any serious injuries to the HSE under RIDDOR (see section 3)</li><li>Inform CQC if any service user has been harmed by the accident</li></ul>
Fire emergency	<ul><li>Raise the alarm.</li><li>Call emergency services.</li><li>Start evacuation procedures (some settings evacuate to another zone within the building).</li><li>Do not use the lift.</li><li>Avoid smoke-filled areas.</li><li>If leaving the building, leave by nearest safe exit.</li><li>Only tackle a fire if safe to do so and you have been trained.</li><li>Assemble at meeting point and do a roll call.</li><li>Write a report of the incident as soon as possible after it has been dealt with.</li></ul>	<ul><li>Call the fire brigade even if the fire has been extinguished.</li><li>Inform CQC if any service users have been harmed.</li><li>Police may be needed if the fire is suspected to be caused by arson.</li></ul>

Incident	Response	Reporting requirements
Flood emergency	• Monitor flood alerts and risk levels. • Prepare for floods by protecting the property with sandbags. • Shut down utilities if possible to reduce damage. • Evacuate service users to higher floors or a different building. • Keep service users and staff up to date with what is happening.	• Liaise with the local authority and social services who have emergency procedures in place for flooding in the area. • Notify CQC if the provision of care in the setting has been impacted. • Record incident reports to allow for review of response.
Chemical or gas leak	• Call emergency services. • Trigger an alert but do not use the fire alarm as it will lead inappropriate responses. • Do not use electrical switches as this could cause an explosion. • Ventilate the building to remove the gas • Remove contaminated clothing as it could cause burns. • Rinse eyes and skin that may have been in contact with the substance (follow risk assessment). • Administer first aid where needed.	• Report to the HSE under RIDDOR if anyone is harmed. • Inform CQC if the wellbeing of any service users have been affected. • Record the incident in an incident log to allow review of polices.
Outbreak of diseases	• Isolate infected individuals to prevent spread of infection. • Implement infection control protocols (such as wearing PPE, enhanced cleaning routine). • Inform staff and service users about the risk. • Seek medical help if necessary.	• Notify the UK Health Security Agency (UKHSA) who need to be informed of outbreaks of disease under RIDDOR. • Inform CQC if service user health and wellbeing has been affected. • Inform social services if it is a care home. • Record incident to enable review of polices.
Missing persons	• Search the building and nearby areas immediately. • Contact the police and report the missing person. • Interview staff and service users to gain more information on where the person might have gone. • People who are likely to go missing should have personalised actions already recorded in their care plan – follow these. • Inform family and other emergency contacts. • Complete the setting's incident report form.	• Report to the police as soon as it is confirmed the person is missing. • Inform CQC. • Contact Social Services if the individual is classed as a vulnerable person. • Use the Herbert Protocol for at-risk adults (provide police with pre-prepared file including a photo, medical information, contacts of the individual and a list of locations they have been known to go regularly).

> **Study Tips!**
> - Knowing the role of the different health and social care settings will help you to identify likely hazards in each setting.
> - You will need to know how different hazards are dealt with in the different settings to reduce the risk that they will cause harm.
> - Remember that hazards can cause harm to staff as well as to service users.
> - The most important part of a risk assessment is applying control measures to reduce the risk caused by the hazards you have identified.
> - You may need to be able to identify ways to respond to health and safety incidents in a given health and social care setting and justify why you have chosen those methods.

Important terms!

Clinical waste – Waste produced from treating individuals. It can include needles and syringes and dressings amongst other things.

Protozoa – A type of microorganism that includes some types that can infect people. Malaria is caused by a protozoan.

Norovirus – A viral infection that causes vomiting and diarrhoea. It is highly contagious and spreads easily through health and social care settings.

Scabies – A skin infection that causes intense itching and a rash with red or brown spots. It is caused by a tiny mite. It can spread easily in health and social care settings.

PPE – Personal protective equipment, designed to protect people from harm. Most forms of PPE are worn such as gloves, aprons, masks and overalls.

Mobile – Where an individual is able to move independently such as walking, repositioning and transferring from a bed to a chair.

Hyperthermia – A condition where the body's core temperature is higher than it should be.

Hypothermia – A condition where the body's core temperature is lower than it should be.

Cross contamination – Where harmful microorganisms that cause infection are transferred from one individual or a surface to another person, causing them to become infected.

Carrier – An individual who has a specific pathogen (or a gene for a disorder) that they can pass on to other people. They may or may not suffer from the disease themselves.

Pressure ulcer – An area of damage to the skin and underlying flesh caused by long periods of pressure on the area. This is often caused by being in a sitting or lying position for a long time without being able to move to relieve the pressure.

CPD – Continuous professional development, which is a requirement for professionals to keep up to date with their learning and development. Professionals need to carry out CPD throughout their careers.

Best practice – The best way of working in health and social care, which takes account of up-to-date legislation, ethical standards, person-centred approaches and research that provides evidence that the intervention works.

Herbert Protocol – An initiative designed to help find vulnerable people with dementia who go missing. It is used by care homes and community settings and helps the police to find the individual quicker.

Recap Questions

1. Define the term 'hazard'.
2. What is the difference between a hazard and a risk?
3. Give an example of a biological hazard in a health and social care setting. Who might be affected by this hazard?
4. Choose a biological hazard. a) What impact can this biological hazard have on people in a hospital ward? b) How can a hospital reduce the risk of this hazard?
5. Why might an X-ray machine pose a hazard to a member of staff in a clinic?
6. What is a risk assessment?
7. Describe a hazard in a hospice which PPE can mitigate against.
8. What are the correct steps to take if a person in care home goes missing?
9. What should the staff in a pharmacy do if a fire breaks out?
10. What is the Health and Safety Executive (HSE)? Which incidents need to be reported to the HSE?
11. What is a control measure?
12. What impact could poor security systems have on a worker in a homeless shelter?
13. Why is staff training in manual handling important in a hospital?

Revision Quiz

1. Give an example of physical abuse that might be seen in a residential care home.
2. What is the difference between an Integrated Care Board (ICB) and Integrated Care Partnership (ICP)?
3. What social impact might neglect have on a child?
4. Why is it important the elderly residents of a care home are treated with dignity?
5. Name two health care setting.
6. What steps could be taken to ensure a same-sex couple are not discriminated against in a maternity ward?
7. A person in a wheelchair is visiting their GP. What reasonable adjustments might the surgery be expected to make?
8. Explain the difference between direct and indirect discrimination and give an example of each.
9. Why is it important for health and social care staff to undergo mandatory training on autism and learning disabilities?
10. What impact might Integrated Care Records have on service users?
11. What impact does the Equality Act have for a same-sex couple on a maternity ward?

Assessment practice

1. Give two possible control measures to reduce the risk of infection. (2)
2. Give three examples of biological hazards that might be found in a nursing home. (3)
3. State two ways the risk from biological hazards can be reduced. (2)
4. State two types of service users who are particularly vulnerable to poor security in a health and social care setting. (2)
5. State two possible consequences of breaking bones in a fall due to poor health and safety (2)
6. Explain what a control measure is. (2)
7. Give three examples of health and safety information that must be displayed clearly in health and social care settings.
8. Give two ways a setting can be kept well maintained to prevent harm. (2)
9. Give three types of emergency situation that might occur in health and social care settings. (3)
10. Describe the need for an accident book in health and social care settings. (3)
11. Explain what a near miss is. (2)
12. Describe reporting procedures to CQC of accidents in the setting. (3)

Mabel was admitted to hospital for hip replacement surgery. In the beginning she recovered well. However, after about a week she had a fever, and her wound showed signs of infection. Antibiotics did not seem to work. She has been diagnosed with MRSA.

13. Explain why poor health and safety at the hospital has caused Mabel to contract MRSA. (3)

A nursing home has been rated by CQC as having poor health and safety record and that staffing levels are too low.

14. Justify why increasing staffing levels could reduce illness, and accidents improve outcomes for service users (6)

St. Michael's Homeless Shelter provides temporary accommodation to individuals and families who are homeless. They have a health and safety policy written when the shelter was open two years ago and it is available in the office for those that need to see it. Risk assessments such as hazards caused by the premises, electrical equipment and cleaning products have all been done. There is a torn carpet in one of the corridors, but all residents have been informed it is there. Wet floor signs are regularly used when the cleaning staff are mopping the bathroom floors. Fire training is carried out every year to train the staff how to act in an emergency and fire exit signs are clear. There is currently an aggressive resident who shouts and threatens staff when he gets drunk. Many of the staff have expressed concerns that they do not know how to deal with this situation. As a result, some staff have left leaving a shortage. However, the manager is helping by carrying out general duties. This leaves them little time for their own duties.

15. Discuss the extent to which the shelter is managing health and safety in the setting. (6)

3: Legislation in health and social care settings

All workplaces and services are required to follow laws devised by the UK government. This legislation applies to everybody in the UK and not just health and social care settings. Some laws are more relevant to health and social care settings than others.

The Equality Act (2010)

Key purpose

It combines all previous equality laws such as those that were for age, disability, race, sex and religion. It also protects groups that were previously not protected by legislation. It sets out 9 protected characteristics:

- Age – protects both younger and older people from age-related discrimination and unfair treatment.
- Disability – this covers all types of disability including physical disabilities, mental impairments, sensory impairments and disabilities due to illness.
- Gender reassignment – protects people who feel they have a different gender to their biological gender from harassment and refusal of service. People are protected regardless of whether they have taken steps to change their gender.
- Marriage and civil partnership – Protects people who are married or who are in a civil partnership.
- Pregnancy and maternity – protects women through their pregnancy, during the birth and postnatal care such as breast feeding.
- Race – protects people from discrimination on the grounds of colour, ethnic group and nationality.
- Religion or belief – protects people who follow a specific religion, and those who do not.
- Sex – protects people from being discriminated against because they are male or female.
- Sexual orientation – protects people from discrimination on the grounds of their sexual preferences.

Main provisions

The law makes it illegal to discriminate against people on the grounds of any of the nine protected characteristics. This includes both direct and indirect discrimination. It also makes harassment and victimisation unlawful.

It is aimed at employers and providers of services including health and social care services.

It requires organisations to make **reasonable adjustments** to be able to offer the same opportunities to everyone regardless of whether they have a protected characteristic or not. Reasonable adjustments are there to overcome barriers that prevent people from accessing work or services.

Impact on service users

- The law ensures equal access to care and support (and employment in health and social care services).
- Protects individuals from unfair treatment in health and social care settings.
- Improves people's trust in health and social care services.
- Ensures dignity for people receiving care.

The Health and Care Act (2022)

Key purpose

- To improve communication and collaboration between the health and the social care sectors. There have been previous instances of serious neglect and abuse that could have been prevented with better working relationships between the two sectors.
- To reduce health inequalities so that everyone should be able to expect the same health outcomes regardless of factors like race or socioeconomic background.
- To reduce delays in care by preventing unnecessary repetition of tasks between the two services.
- To improve local planning of services and workforce to be better able to meet the needs of the local community.

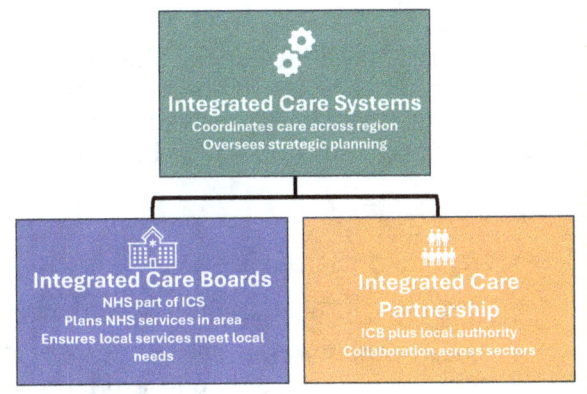

Main provisions

- Created **Integrated Care Systems (ICS)**.
  - » **Integrated Care Boards (ICBs)** which plan NHS services locally.
  - » **Integrated Care Partnerships (ICPs)** to create long-term plans to support the health and wellbeing of the population of the area. Prevention of illness is a key focus.

  These Integrated Care Services involve professionals across NHS, local authorities, charities, mental health services and service users themselves.
- Introduced **advertising restrictions** of less healthy food and drink which includes:
  - » Banning advertising of high-fat, high-sugar food or drink between 5.30am and 9pm on TV and on-demand platforms.
  - » Ban such advertising on social media and websites at all times.
- Shared health and social care records to prevent unnecessary repetition and to improve communication. It does this by introducing **Integrated Care Records (ICRs)** which are shared records used by GPs, hospitals and social services.
- Introduced **data sharing requirements** by making it a requirement to share data about health such as cancer rates and data about people receiving social care services. This information is handled securely without revealing details about individual people.
  - » The data is managed by the **Health and Social Care Information Centre (HSCIC).** The information helps plan appropriate services.
- Allowed some **social care needs assessments** to be **carried out after the individual has been discharged** from hospital so long as they are discharged to somewhere safe such as a care home and where no new care needs have arisen. This prevents bed-blocking.
- **Banned virginity testing** and makes it a criminal offense to perform, arrange or assist in virginity testing even if the individual has consented. The ban applies to UK citizens both in the UK and abroad to prevent people being sent out of the country to have the test.
- Makes it mandatory for everyone working in health and social care, including admin and auxiliary staff of CQC regulated settings, to **complete training on learning disabilities and autism**.

Impact on service users

- Reduces delays for service users to receive care and support.
- Ensures that the support provided is holistic, taking account of all their needs.
- Improves public health overall to reduce the pressure on health and social care services.
- Makes it easier for health and social care providers to plan for example ensuring they recruit enough staff and specialists.
- Makes it easier to clear hospital beds for new patients
- Reduces duplication so that service users do not have to answer the same questions for different services.

The Children Act (2004)

Key purpose

The Children Act was introduced after the death of Victoria Climbié and the Laming report that was produced as a result. Its aim is to protect children who are at risk of harm and promote children's rights, wellbeing and enable them to participate in decisions made about their lives. It aimed to strengthen cooperation between agencies to safeguard children more effectively.

Main provisions

- Protects children from harm by:
  - Requiring local authorities to work with other agencies to safeguard children.
  - Local authorities must also set up **Local Safeguarding Children Boards (LSCBs)** to coordinate safeguarding investigations.
- The paramountcy principle:
  - When services have any involvement with children, the **needs of the child must be paramount** (the primary concern) and should be taken into account for all decisions.
  - The paramountcy principle applies to courts, social services, schools and care providers.
- The right to be consulted:
  - Children must be given the opportunity to **express their views about decisions** that affect them. This does not mean that they will be the only one making decision about themselves.
  - Methods used to involve children in decision making will depend on their age. Play can be used for younger children.
  - The view of older children, particularly adolescents, will carry more weight.
- Right to an **advocate** to help children speak up for themselves. The advocate can be independent (must not represent any of the agencies involved in the decision) or could be a parent or other relative.
- Requires **partnership working** e.g. between health services, social care, education, the police and families. It involves sharing of information, carrying out joint assessments and making decisions together as a team.
- Introduces the role of **Children's Commissioner** who:
  - Promotes the rights and interests of children
  - Gathers views of children so that services can be better tailored to their needs
  - Supports initiatives such as The Big Ask, Help at Hand and In My Opinion (IMO).

Impact on service users

- Improves protection of children from harm and abuse.
- Gives children a voice in decisions that affect them.
- Gives a right to advocacy so children do not feel alone.
- Coordinated services are less likely to miss signs of abuse.
- Sharing information reduces opportunities for abuse and improves services.
- Safeguarding boards ensure that organisations learn about what can go wrong so they can prevent it happening in the future.

Data Protection Act 2018 (GDPR)

Key purpose

The Data Protection Act of 2018, which covers the General Data Protection Regulations, built on previous legislation to protect people's individual data and included provision for online data. Its aim is to safeguard personal data and ensure the right to privacy of information. It provides clear rules for how organisations, including health and social care settings, should handle, store and share information.

Main provisions

The law sets out seven core principles:

1. **Lawfulness, fairness and transparency** – includes the requirement to obtain consent to hold data about a person, the need to be clear about what the data is held for and not being able to use data without permission.

2. **Purpose limitation** – organisations can only collect data for clearly defined reasons and the data cannot be reused for something else (such as be sold to companies who want to sell you something). It requires that if data is used for research, the data is anonymised.

3. **Data minimisation** – only necessary and relevant information should be collected to avoid excessive data collection. If information is not needed in order to provide the service, it should not be collected.

4. **Accuracy** – data should be correct and up to date. Individuals have a right to see the data and have it corrected if it is wrong. Organisations must regularly review the data they hold.

5. **Storage limitation** – data must not be used for longer than is required which is likely to be:
   » Medical records are typically kept for 7-10 years
   » Employment records for 6-10 years after the end of the employment
   » Some records, such as child protection records, are kept permanently

6. **Integrity and confidentiality** – data must be stored securely and only shared with authorised individuals. IT systems must be in place to protect digital data and these must be updated regularly. Staff need to receive training on confidentiality and organisations must have protocols to follow if there is a breach of data.

7. **Accountability** – organisations need to demonstrate they have adequate systems for protecting data. They must appoint a Data Protection Officer (DPO) who:
   » Is responsible for data within the organisation.
   » Monitors security systems.
   » Ensures there are procedures on ensuring people are asked their consent to hold data about them.
   » Ensures that other organisations they work with have adequate data protection.

Impact on service users

- Service users have greater control over the information held about them by organisations.
- Service users and staff are clear about what data is held about them and what it is used for.
- Individuals have the right to see what information an organisation is holding about them.
- Service users can have more confidence in the safety of their data.
- Care practitioners and organisations have clear rules about the storage, handling and use of data.
- Having a DPO makes it more likely that data rules will be followed and ensures people know who to turn to when they have concerns or questions.

Health and Safety at Work Act (1974)

Key purpose

The aim is to ensure safety for employees at work. It makes employers legally responsible for health and safety in their organisation. However, it also requires that employers take responsibility for their own health and safety so they have to comply with procedures.

Main provisions

Employer responsibilities include:

- Must create and maintain health and safety policies.
- Must carry out risk assessments to reduce the risk of harm.
- Ensure that the physical environment and equipment used is safe.
- Must ensure security of the setting.
- Provide adequate training to staff on health and safety procedures.
- Must provide PPE and equipment to ensure safety of staff and service users.
- Must consult employees and service users about health and safety matters.
- Must make sure first aid arrangements are in place.

Employee responsibilities:

- Must follow risk assessments.
- Must attend training and apply what they have learned.
- Must use equipment correctly and safely.
- Must report accidents and faulty equipment.
- Must not behave in a way that puts themselves or others at risk of harm.

Impact on service users

- Ensures a safe environment for service users, staff and others such as visitors.
- Increases service user's confidence in services.
- Increases confidence of staff are they have the training and procedures so that they know what is expected of them and how to work safely.
- Requirements to keep health and safety records ensures that actions can be tracked and services can be improved in relation to health and safety.
- Safer workplaces promote staff retention.

Manual Handling Operations Regulations (1992)

Key purpose

This legislation is an addition to the Health and Safety at Work Act, with specific relevant to moving and handling loads and people. Its main aim is to reduce injuries caused by lifting, carrying, pushing and pulling objects or people at work. The requirements also protect the service users who are going to be moved.

Main provisions

- **Avoid unnecessary manual handling** where possible. This could be by eliminating the tasks, reducing the need to lift or carry such as by using hoists and hand trucks.
- **Assess the risks of the procedure** for each different manual handling task considering the following:
  » The load (or person) being moved such as weight, stability, unpredictability and their willingness and ability to assist
  » Staff capability including fitness and other conditions such as pregnancy
  » The environment such as whether there is clutter, how much space there is and where there are trip hazards
- Reduce the risk of injury by **setting out what the task requires** which may include:
  » Moving furniture out of the way before carrying out the move.
  » Use specific equipment like hoists, slide sheets, transfer boards and adjustable beds.
  » Ensure enough staff are available for the task – manual handling of people often requires two members of staff.
  » Take account of the health needs of staff carrying out the task – pregnant women are often not allowed to move and handle people to protect them from injury.
  » Ensure that there are sufficient breaks during intensive moving and handling.
- **Provide training and supervision** to ensure all staff carry out procedures safely and correctly and know how to protect themselves from harm by having the right posture and techniques. Employers have a duty to provide information, training and supervision.

Impact on service users

- Service users will be moved in a safe and comfortable way and will have more trust in the service.
- The risk of injuries to both service users and staff with be reduced.
- Service users will be moved in a way that is personalised to their individual needs.
- Staff sickness due to musculoskeletal problems should be reduced.

Control of Substances Hazardous to Health (COSHH) (2002)

Key purpose

COSHH aims to protect service users, staff and others from harm caused by hazardous substances which include:

- Chemicals
- Cleaning agents
- Medicines
- Bodily fluids
- Fumes
- Gases
- Dust
- Biological agents such as bacteria and viruses

Main provisions

The organisation must carry out risk assessments on all substances that will be used or will be found in the setting. They need to hold specific information about the substances and reduce the risk of harm. The main provisions of the legislation are as follows:

- **Prevent or reduce exposure** to hazardous substances by:
  » Removing hazardous substances where possible.
  » Substituting dangerous chemicals for safer alternatives.
  » Use PPE when working with these substances to reduce exposure.
  » Isolated infected patients to minimise the spread of infectious agents.
  » Keep areas where fumes may build up, such as cleaning cupboards, well ventilated.
  » Have clear protocols for labelling, storage and disposal of hazardous substances
- **Store, label and dispose of substances safely**:
  » Store hazardous substances such as cleaning products in locked rooms that have signs to indicate that substances are stored there.
  » Use specialist bins to dispose of clinical waste – clinical waste bins which are disposed of by a licensed specialist company.
  » Controlled medication needs to be signed off by two members of staff for enhanced security.
  » Never transfer substances to unlabelled containers or into a container that is labelled for something else.
  » Follow requirements for temperature and ventilation when storing chemicals including cleaning products.
- **Staff training is mandatory** for all staff working in health and social care and covers COSHH awareness, safe handling and disposal of substances, equipment needed, how to reduce risk form substances and emergency procedures such as when there is a chemical spill.
- **Keep an up-to-date COSHH file** on the premises to include all the COSHH risk assessments for each substance. The COSHH risk assessment includes:
  » Health effects of exposure to the substance.
  » Any PPE requirements when working with the substance.
  » Emergency procedures to follow if exposed to the substance.
- The **risk assessments should be reviewed annually** or more often if circumstances change.

Impact on service users

- Lower risk of harm to service users, staff and others such as visitors.
- Environments are safer for vulnerable groups such as those with dementia who may not understand the risks.
- Organisations have a clear guide on how to handle and store each substance, what information to keep about them and what to do in case of an emergency.

Reporting of Injuries, Diseases and Dangerous Occurrences Regulations (RIDDOR) (2013)

Key purpose

Ensures that all serious incidents, illnesses and near misses in health and social care settings are reported to the appropriate authorities so that action can be taken if settings are not doing enough to protect people. The Health and Safety Executive (HSE) uses the information to track trends so that they can target safety interventions.

Main provisions

- Organisations are **required to keep records of incidents** as follows:
    » Internal records (such as an accident book) for all injuries to service users and staff and incidents that could have caused harm but by luck did not (these are near misses).
    » Report to HSE for injuries to staff that means they are off work for 7 or more consecutive days, accidents that caused fractures (except to the fingers, thumbs and toes), injuries that lead to amputation of limbs, burns covering 10% or more of the body and permanent blindness. The following incidents must also be reported: collapsing hoists, spills of hazardous materials, explosions and major equipment failure.
- Use an **accident book** within the setting for all accidents. These records include:
    » Date and time of incident and details of people involved
    » Description of the injury and the actions taken following the injury
    » Details of any witnesses to the incident
    » Any follow-up steps taken
- The accident book should be used to **track trends within the setting** to review procedures and improve safety
- **Report listed diseases to the UK Health Security Agency (UKHSE)** who use it to track the spread of harmful diseases. Reportable illnesses include, amongst others:
    » Hepatitis A, B and C
    » Tuberculosis
    » Covid-19
    » Legionnaire's disease
    » Measles
    » Acute meningitis.

Impact on service users

- Reporting diseases improves response time of the authorities so they can reduce the spread of dangerous diseases.
- The legislation requires organisations and the HSE to track trends in accidents and incidents so that underlying causes can be removed and safety improved.
- Service users, staff and others will be reduced to fewer hazardous situations.
- Helps organisations to make safety improvements.
- Organisations are held accountable for health and safety within their settings.

Study Tips!
- You will need to know how each law supports individual rights, provides guidance and is used as a framework for running the health and social care service.
- You can help memorise the 9 characteristics of the Equality Act by remembering the name Dr Grampss (remember the double S). D – disability, R – race, G – gender reassignment, R – religion or belief, A – age, M – marriage and civil partnership, P – pregnancy and maternity, S – sex, S- sexual orientation.

> **Important terms!**
>
> **Civil partnership** – A legal partnership between two people giving similar rights to being married. It is usually associated with same-sex couples, but mixed sex couples can also get a civil partnership.
>
> **Health inequalities** – Where some groups of people in society suffer more illnesses or even die younger, and have less access to healthcare than other groups.
>
> **Bed-blocking** – When a patient is occupying a hospital bed only because they have nowhere safe to be discharged to. Their medical needs have been met as far as they can be within the hospital, so they do not actually need hospital care.
>
> **Holistic care** – Care and support that takes the whole person into consideration rather than just focusing on their disorder or condition they might have. It considers the person such as their physical, intellectual, emotional, social and financial priorities.
>
> **Slide sheet** – A slippery sheet that is placed under an individual to be able to move them easily into the right position. They are usually folded into a tube so that two sheets slide against each other.
>
> **Transfer board** – A board used to transfer a person from one place to another such as from one chair to another or across from one bed to another. The individual slides or is slid across the board.
>
> **Controlled medication** – Medicines that have extra controls on them because they are at a higher risk of being misused. Morphine is an example of a controlled medication.
>
> **Near miss** – An incident that could have caused harm but didn't just because of luck. Near misses need to be taken as seriously as accidents because next time it might cause an injury.

Recap Questions

1. How does the Equality Act protect disabled service users of health and social care settings?
2. What is a 'protected characteristic' under the Equality Act?
3. What is an Integrated Care Board (ICB)?
4. What is virginity testing?
5. Which Act required data to be shared across different services?
6. What is the impact of advertising restrictions on high-fat high-sugar foods?
7. What is the paramountcy principle?
8. How does the Children's Act aim to protect children from harm?
9. What does the Children's Commissioner do?
10. What does data minimisation mean?
11. What impact does GDPR have for people who visit an optician?
12. A GP surgery is contacting all of its patients. What does it mean for it to be 'transparent' about its use of patient data?
13. What are two employer responsibilities under the Health and Safety at Work Act?
14. What are two employee responsibilities under the Health and Safety at Work Act?
15. What is 'manual handling'?
16. What are two ways to reduce the risks associated with manual handling?
17. Give two examples of substances in a hospital that are hazardous to human health.
18. What is controlled medication?
19. What must be recorded in an Accident Book?
20. What needs to be reported to the UK Health Security Agency under RIDDOR? Give one example.

Revision Quiz

1. How might staff meetings help health care workers apply best practice?
2. Why might a hazard in a hospital lead to financial loss?
3. What does disclosure mean?
4. How might young people experience discrimination in a health care setting?
5. What is a blended family?
6. Why might lack of adequate supervision of staff in a day centre be a potential hazard?
7. Name an incident that must be reported to the CQC.
8. Give two examples of discriminatory behaviour in a hospital.
9. What are the five rights that every individual has in a health and social care setting?
10. What is meant by the term 'clinical waste?'
11. Give an example of age discrimination in a hospital.
12. What does the term 'socio-economic background' mean?
13. What impact might disempowerment have on a young person with learning disabilities?

Assessment practice

1. Describe what is meant by direct discrimination. (1)
2. Give two examples of indirect discrimination towards users of health and social care services. (2)
3. State two systems brought in by the Health and Care Act 2022 to help health and social care services to work better together. (2)
4. State the name of the shared health and social care record. (1)
5. Describe the criminality of virginity testing under the Health and Care Act 2022 (3)
6. Give the name of the report which triggered the Children Act 2004 to be created. (1)
7. State the name of the boards that local authorities are required to set up under the act. (1)
8. State the names of two initiatives used by the Children's Commissioner to gather the views of children. (2)
9. State three of the seven principles of the Data Protection Act. (3)
10. Give three pieces of information if might be relevant to collect about an individual receiving healthcare services. (3)
11. State the name of the role that must be allocated to someone in organisations to ensure accountability of information. (1)
12. Give three examples of an employer's responsibilities under the Health and Safety at Work Act 1974. (3)

13. Choose which of the following are responsibilities for people who work in health and social care services. (3)

    A   Decide based on the situation as to whether to follow the risk assessment or not.
    B   Use equipment as it was intended to be used.
    C   Attend training on health and safety and put the learning into practice.
    D   They may have to take risks to protect other people such as catching a service user who is falling.
    E   Behave sensibly.

14. State the first and most important way or preventing harm due to moving and handling. (1)

15. State three things that are likely to be covered on moving and handling training in health and social care settings. (3)

16. State three different types of substances that COSHH might relate to. (3)

17. Give two things covered in COSHH training. (2)

18. Describe the requirement under the act on keeping information of hazardous substances that are found in the setting. (3)

19. Give the name of the organisation to which accidents must be reported under RIDDOR. (1)

20. Choose which of the following should be reported under RIDDOR. (3)

    A   Burns covering more than 10% of the body.
    B   A broken finger.
    C   That a worker has fallen and had to be off work for the rest of the day.
    D   An accident involving a hoist.
    E   A chemical burn.

4: Best practice in health and social care settings

4.1 Person-centred values

Person-centred care puts the individual at the heart of the service and at the heart of every decision. This makes the support they receive more likely to fit their needs, values, beliefs and wishes rather than just being imposed on them. The service user becomes a vital member of the team.

- **Applying person-centred values** ensures all needs are met and that the individual feels supported. This will speed recovery from illnesses as wellbeing has a big impact on this. The service user will have greater trust and confidence in the service. The individual feels like they are a person who is values and respected rather than just someone else's work.

- **Failing to promote person-centred values** can have serious consequences. It will have a negative impact on the health of the individual. It can impact their mental health because the individual may feel powerless in their own life. Reduced trust in services may lead to the individual not heeding health advice, leading to poor health outcomes. There are nine person-centred values that are set out in the table below.

Value	How it is promoted in practice
Individuality	Service users must be treated as an individual with their differences acknowledged and accepted. Support should take account of their different needs and wishes. Specific examples: • Important information about the individual is recorded in a care plan. • Assessments look at the whole person not just their condition and combine health and social care needs. • Services are more accessible (such as extended opening hours) to meet individual needs. • Preferences and beliefs are taken into account when planning the support.
Choice	Giving people choice gives them control over their lives. • Clear information about treatments and support options is given so the individual can make an informed choice. • Choice is offered where possible including choice of food, choice of appointment times, choice of activity etc. • Families and advocates can be involved in helping make choices if the individual is unable to do so themselves.
Rights	Supporting rights means people are treated with dignity and respect and that their needs are met. The requirement to uphold rights is stated in the Human Rights Act and Equality Act and in codes of practice for health and social care professionals. • Treatments and care must be agreed to before being carried out, so consent must be gained. • Data should be handled with care as per the Data Protection Act. • Advocates can be used to help individuals express their views so that they can have their rights upheld.
Independence	Independence means being able to do as much for yourself as possible. Losing independence increases reliance on others and reduces choice and emotional wellbeing. • Adapt self-care tasks so the individual can do more of it themselves, such as clothes that are easier to put on. • Use technology to assist the individual such as pill organisers. • Rehabilitation services can help service users regain lost skills. • Life skills training programmes can help teach people to be more independent.

Value	How it is promoted in practice
Privacy	Privacy relates to an individual's body, information held about them, conversations they have and their personal space. Health and social care workers should not intrude on someone's privacy without consent. • Knock and wait for an answer before entering someone's room. • Use consulting rooms with privacy curtains for treatments. • Allow private areas for visits in care settings. • Ensure dignity when someone has to get undressed e.g. for an MRI scan – robes should be available.
Dignity	Dignity is treating the person as a valued individual, listening to them and respecting them. Not treating someone with dignity impacts their self-esteem and improves their trust in the service. • When assisting someone to wash, only uncover the part being washed at that moment. • Use someone's preferred name and pronoun. • Provide support without showing any judgement. • Show compassion during assessments and treatments.
Respect	Respecting someone means valuing them as an individual and recognising their rights. • Use preferred names and pronouns. • Pay full attention during conversations. • Never use a mobile phone when you are supposed to be listening to them. • Settings should offer culturally sensitive space for prayer. • Services should be fair and inclusive to all regardless of any protected characteristics they might have.
Partnership	The individual (and their family if that is what they want) should be treated as partners in the support team. They should be fully involved in all decisions about their care, support and treatment.
Encouraging service users' decision making	For some service users more support will be needed to encourage or enable them to make decisions about themselves. Information may need to be broken down or the format changed so that they understand what they are deciding about.

4.2 The 6Cs

The 6Cs are all values beginning with the letter C that health and social care workers should hold. Together they ensure service users are treated with dignity and respect, and they get the best possible service. The 6Cs are as follows:

- **Care** – health and social care workers should care about the individual including treating them as an individual, with respect and dignity.
- **Compassion** – workers should develop a connection with the individual and understand the situation from the point of view of the service user.
- **Competence** – workers should have the skills and knowledge to be able to do their job properly.
- **Communication** – workers should have good communication skills and be able to adapt their communication to the needs and abilities of the service users.
- **Courage** – workers should have the mental strength to do what is right even when other people disagree. They also need to have the courage to tell service users the truth about their situation rather than what they want to hear.
- **Commitment** – workers need to be determined to provide the best service to people. They must be prepared to learn from mistakes, keep up to date with training and constantly improve.

Some examples of the 6Cs in specific settings:

6Cs	Examples in practice
Care	- Hospices support families during end-of-life care. - Pharmacies offer advice on minor illnesses. - Food banks provide essentials to those in financial crisis.
Compassion	- Dental services use calming techniques for anxious patients to improve the experience of the treatment. - Homeless shelters welcome individuals without judgement. - Mobile screening unit staff explain results of test with sensitivity.
Competence	- GPs give accurate diagnoses due to their knowledge and experience which will improve outcomes for service users. - Hospice staff provide skilled end-of-life support to maintain dignity and comfort of the individual. - Social workers discuss tailored care options to allow service users to make the most appropriate decisions for them.
Communication	- Social care services use visual aids and simple language where needed to aid communication. - Workers interpret non-verbal cues such as a service user wandering the corridors may mean they need the toilet. - Support groups create safe spaces by using strict confidentiality rules.
Courage	- Reporting unsafe colleague behaviour to protect service users even if they are friendly with the colleague. - Social workers make tough safeguarding decisions such as putting a child into temporary care to protect them from abuse. - Emergency teams respond to critical, unpredictable events which can be frightening.
Commitment	- Workers undertake CPD to keep up to date with the latest best practice. - Workers stay beyond their finishing time, where needed, to support an individual during a critical stage in their treatment.

4.3 Safeguarding in health and social care settings

Safeguarding is the policies, procedures and practices used by services to protect the health and wellbeing of the individuals within their care. Safeguarding is relevant to both children and adults. All health and social care settings have a safeguarding duty. Effective safeguarding not only responds to harm and abuse but aims to prevent it as well by empowering individuals to speak up.

Safeguarding policies in care settings

Care settings are required to have robust safeguarding policies and procedures by the Health and Care Act 2022. These guide staff on how to recognise, report and respond to concerns. They emphasise the importance of collaboration with other agencies to ensure the individual is protected. Safeguarding policies are for children and vulnerable adults.

Aims of safeguarding policies

- To stop abuse and neglect of individuals who use the service.
- Prevent harm including from accidents and illness.
- Reduce the likelihood that service users will be abused or neglected by making it easier for staff to spot warning signs and making it easier for service users to report their concerns.
- Acknowledging that vulnerable adults have a right to live their life how they want and so supports them in making choices and giving them control over their life.

Key features of the policy

- Each setting should appoint a **designated safeguarding lead (DSL)**. The DSL has overall responsibility for safeguarding in the setting. They can advise other staff on actions to take and they ensure that procedures are followed.
- **Training** on safeguarding should be given to all staff and updated regularly. Staff who do not provide direct care such as cleaning staff must also undertake the training. The policy will set out what type of training each level of staff must have and how often it should be repeated.
- Anyone who works with children or vulnerable adults must first have a **DBS check.** DBS stands for disclosure and barring.
    - » The check looks to see if the potential staff member has any convictions and can also check if they have been added to the list of people who are barred from working with children or vulnerable adults.
    - » Workers who have direct contact with service users must have an enhanced DBS check. Those who work in health and social care settings but without direct contact (such as administrative staff) can have a standard DBS check.

People who may need safeguarding

Knowing who might be at risk of abuse, neglect or exploitation will make health and social care workers more vigilant to warning signs. They can also help to prevent abuse. Some groups of people are more likely to be abused (vulnerable groups). This could be because they are less likely to resist, less likely to be believed or even less likely to know that they are being abused.

Group	Details
Children	- Less able to protect themselves due to being physically weaker. - Dependent on their carers so they could worry about being abandoned. - May not understand that what they are experiencing is abuse. - Tend to be less confident talking to adults so less likely to report the abuse.
People in residential care settings	- Depend on others for daily support and so may fear they will not get the support they need if they report abuse. - People who require support are more likely to be mistreated in institutional settings by the workers. - Some settings develop a culture of abuse. - Some may have cognitive impairments making it harder for them to recognise and report abuse.
People with physical or learning disabilities	- People with physical disabilities are less able to physically defend themselves so are more likely to be targeted. - People with learning disabilities may not understand that they are being abused. - People with learning disabilities may have communication difficulties that makes it harder for them to report abuse. - Both groups are more dependent on others making them more likely to be abused.
People with mental health conditions	- May lack confidence and emotional resilience to report concerns. - More likely to be socially isolated making them more vulnerable. - They may not be believed if they reported the abuse.
People with sensory impairments	- May be reliant on others who could exploit them in a way they would not notice. - They may fear losing the care support if they reported abuse.
People dependent on carers	- There is a power imbalance between the carer and service user. - Carers may be under stress and overworked so more likely to take out their frustrations on the service user or be rough to save time. - Abuse is more likely in settings where poor practice is tolerated.

Impacts of lack of safeguarding

Physical	Bruises, broken or deformed bones, burn marks, malnourishment, poor growth in children, pregnancy, sexually transmitted diseases, permanent damage to sexual organs.
Intellectual	Difficulty concentrating, poor school performance, difficulty managing day-to-day lives, cognitive decline and risk of dementia.
Emotional	Depression, anxiety, nightmares, low self-esteem, shame, difficulty coping with everyday life.
Social	Isolation and withdrawal, difficulty forming relationships, fear of disclosure, lack of trust.

Dealing with disclosures

Disclosure is when someone shares that abuse has taken place.

- Anyone can disclose abuse including the victim, a witness or even the person who carried out the abuse.
- There should be detailed procedures of what to do if someone discloses abuse to you.
- It will also be covered in the mandatory safeguarding training.
- Health and social care workers **must** report any abuse even if the victim asks them not to – it is a legal duty.

Some types of abuse include:

Type of abuse	Examples
Physical	Causing physical harm by: hitting, kicking, biting, burning, restraining, denying food or medical help.
Emotional	Treating someone in a way that lowers their self-esteem and self-worth including insulting, intimidating, isolating or gaslighting them.
Sexual	Forcing or coercing someone to take part in any type of unwanted sexual behaviour. Children and adults and both males and females can be victims. It can include touching, sexual language and making sexual suggestions, forcing them to look at sexual images, and rape. Sex with someone under the age of 16 is rape.
Neglect	Where the carer does not provide proper care and protection to the individual. It includes not providing food or drink, not providing appropriate and clean clothing, ignoring or not providing emotional support, leaving them alone for long periods, not allowing a child to have an education.
Financial	Controlling someone's money or property. It can include coercing or tricking someone to leave money in their will, stealing money or valuables, conning someone out of money such as by tricking them to pay for unnecessary services.

Requirements of people who work in health and social care

- Follow safeguarding procedures with regard to reporting abuse.
- Report to the DSL on the same day as the disclosure.
- Create a clear written or electronic record of the disclosure.
- Use the individual's own words in the report to avoid misunderstandings.
- Include the names of people involved including victim, alleged abuser and any witnesses.
- Record what actions have been taken.
- Support the individual.
- Provide a safe place for them to speak to you freely.
- Offer comfort and reassurance but do not make promises you cannot keep.
- Inform them that you need to report the abuse as you have a duty to do so.
- Avoid judging the victim or blaming them for the abuse
- Reassure them that confidentiality will be kept as far as possible
- Maintain confidentiality
- Only share information about the abuse to those that need to know, such as the DSL. Do not share automatically with colleagues.
- Follow the Data Protection Act 2018 with regard to keeping information safe
- Protect yourself
- Be aware that you may be at risk from the perpetrator of the abuse and take precautions
- Receiving a disclosure can be emotionally difficult so seek support when needed
- Share your feelings about the disclosure in supervision meetings with your manager or with the DSL
- Protect yourself from accusations of wrongdoing by following the procedures on dealing with disclosures

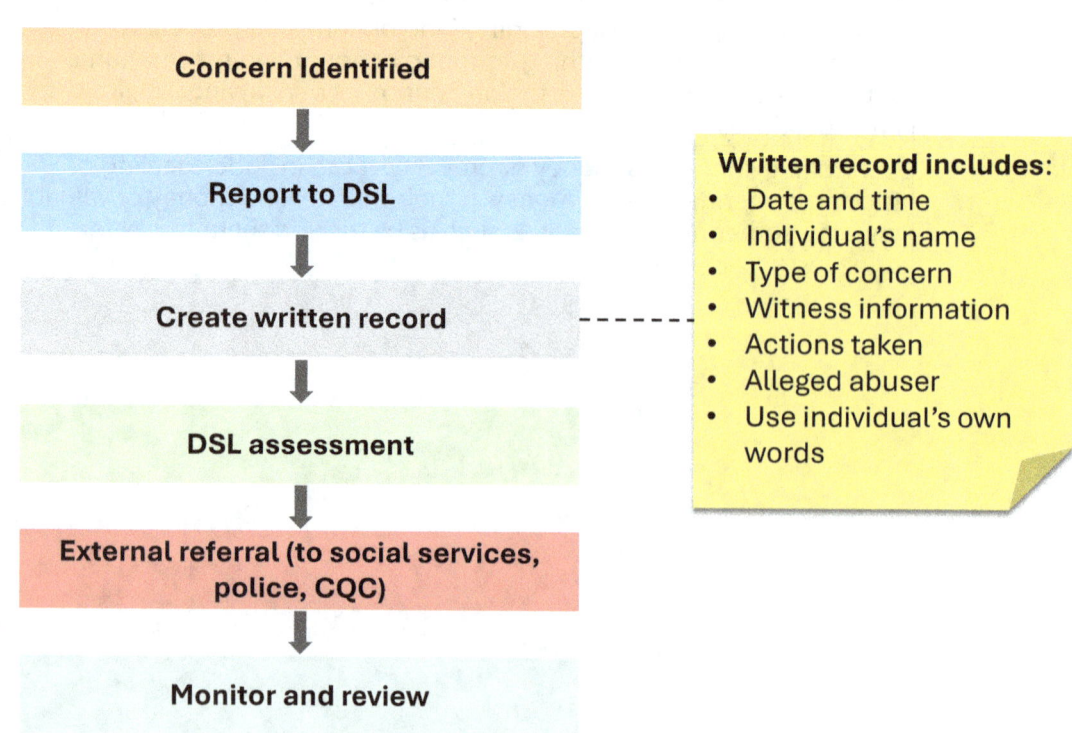

4.4 Supporting practitioners to apply best practice in health and social care settings

Best practice is a term used in health and social care and relates to using the most effective and up-to-date methods that have evidence to show that they work (evidence-based). Best practice takes account of all relevant legislation, research into the particular area, any new technology that has been developed for that area of health or care.

Benefits of best practice include:

- **Service users** – receive high-quality care that is tailored to their needs and is more likely to be effective.
- **Health and social care workers** – will feel competent because they know their ways of working have been checked.
- **Health and social care services** – will achieve better outcomes for their service users which will help them gain a good reputation.

Some of the aspects of best practice are covered below.

Effective communication

- Good communication between health and social care workers and the management is vital
- Workers must be informed when legislation or procedures have changed or they won't know to change how they work
- Communication should be a two-way process so that workers feel they can discuss concerns and difficulties with ways of working
- There should be mechanisms for health and social care staff to feedback to managers about issues that affect their ability to do their jobs to their best ability
- Communication should be supportive

Training and professional development

Training needs to be regular, accessible and relevant to the job the worker is doing. It can include new legislation, how to manage a particular condition, how to use digital tools and many more.

Why it matters	How to support it
Keeps health and social care workers up to date with the latest best practice guidelines	CPD opportunities should be offered, and staff must be given time off to attend the training
Can boost career progression and motivation which will help retain staff and ensure they work well.	Training can be linked to promotion pathways
Increases the skill sets of the health and social care workers so they are better able to meet the needs of service users in a way that maintains their dignity.	Some training should relate to specific skills. Refresher training should be offered where relevant such as for safeguarding training.

Mentoring, monitoring and performance management

Mentoring, monitoring and performance management should be supportive so that the health and social care worker feels safe to express any concerns or difficulties they are having.

- **Mentoring** is usually provided by more experienced colleagues and can involve showing them how to do a specific task as well as providing advice on procedures
- **Monitoring** is carried out by the worker's line manager within the setting. They will monitor standards and suggest CPD opportunities. Many practitioners are also responsible to professional bodies such as the Nursing and Midwifery Council (NMC) who will monitor that they have the right skills and provide a code of conduct for them to work to.
- **Performance management** is carried out by the line manager. It involves annual performance reviews where strengths and weaknesses are identified and a plan is devised to build on the strengths and address any weaknesses. Performance management also involves the line manager carrying out disciplinary or capability procedures if the staff member is not working as well as they should.

Staff meetings to discuss best practice

Staff meetings help workers to talk through problems that affect their work and come up with shared solutions. They should be held regularly and encourage shared learning. Effective meetings will build the workers into an effective team and reinforce high expectations and standards.

Study Tips!
- You may need to identify what values are being demonstrated in a scenario.
- You need to understand the importance of applying best practice from the point of view of service users, practitioners and providers.

Important terms!

Enhanced DBS check – A criminal record check that includes spent and unspent convictions, cautions and other information from local police.

Standard DBS check – A criminal record check that has less information than an enhanced check but still includes spent and unspent convictions, cautions, reprimands and warnings.

Gaslighting – A type of psychological manipulation where someone makes someone else doubt themselves, including doubting their memory, perception of events or sanity.

Supervision meetings – Regular one-to-one meetings between the health or social care practitioner and their line manager or other relevant professional. The aim is to review performance, provide support and identify development needs.

Line manager – An individual that directly manages you without necessarily being the highest manager. Many line managers are managed by someone in a higher position than them.

Disciplinary procedure – A formal process used to address misconduct or inappropriate behaviour. If the misconduct was not bad enough to warrant immediate dismissal, the disciplinary procedure aims to support the individual to improve.

Capability procedure – A process to help improve the performance of a worker who is not working as well as they should. It could include extra support and training as well as targets for improvement.

Recap Questions

1. In terms of person-centred care, define the terms 'dignity' and 'respect'.
2. Why is independence an important value for someone attending a day centre?
3. Name two other person-centred values.
4. What does it mean to treat a service user with 'compassion'?
5. Name two more of the 6Cs.
6. Why are the 6Cs important?
7. What is the aim of safeguarding?
8. What is a Designated Safeguarding Lead?
9. Why do staff working in a children's residential home require a DBS check?
10. Why do people with learning disabilities require safeguarding?
11. What might be the emotional impact of a lack of safeguarding in a care home?
12. Define the term 'sexual abuse'.
13. Why might people receiving domiciliary care be at risk of financial abuse?
14. Give an example of best practice for a manager of a homeless shelter.

Revision Quiz

1. a) Name all of the person-centred values of care. b) Explain why you think the person-centred values of care are important.
2. Give an example of a neurological disorder.
3. What is an infectious disease?
4. What is a health and safety policy and procedure?
5. How might a person's clothes be influenced by their culture?
6. What impact could noise have on service users in a hospice?
7. Explain the difference between ethnicity and race.
8. Why is it important for a care home to understand the cultural identity of its residents?
9. What is the Herbert Protocol?
10. What is an Integrated Care Partnership (ICP)?

Assessment practice

1. Explain what promoting individuality means. (2)
2. Explain how providing information about treatment options promotes choice. (2)
3. Choose the three best methods of promoting independence for someone with mobility problems:
    - A Take them in a wheelchair to where they want to go so, they have more time to do the activity they enjoy.
    - B Support them to walk by themselves with assistance if they can.
    - C Use equipment to help the individual do as much for themselves as possible.
    - D Strongly encourage them to walk even if they feel tired and not up to it today.
    - E Follow the care plan.
4. Describe two ways of helping individuals to make a decision about their care. (2)
5. In relation to the 6Cs, explain the meaning of competence. (1)
6. State three ways commitment can be shown in health and social care services. (2)
7. Give three aims of the safeguarding policy. (3)
8. State the two things a DBS checks about an individual. (2)
9. State one intellectual impact of abuse on children. (1)
10. Explain what a disclosure of abuse is. (1)
11. Give two examples of financial abuse. (2)
12. State three things a report of suspected abuse will include. (3)
13. Explain why good communication within a setting helps ensure best practice. (1)
14. Give two reasons why continuous training and development will help support best practice. (2)
15. State two sources of performance management for health and social care professionals. (2)

Unit F091: Anatomy and physiology for health and social

1: Cardiovascular system

1.1 Composition and function of blood

White blood cells

White blood cells make up **less than 1% of the volume of blood**.

Functions of white blood cells:
- To fight infections.
- By producing antibodies.
- **Phagocytosis** (engulfing and destroying the pathogen).
- To destroy cancer cells.

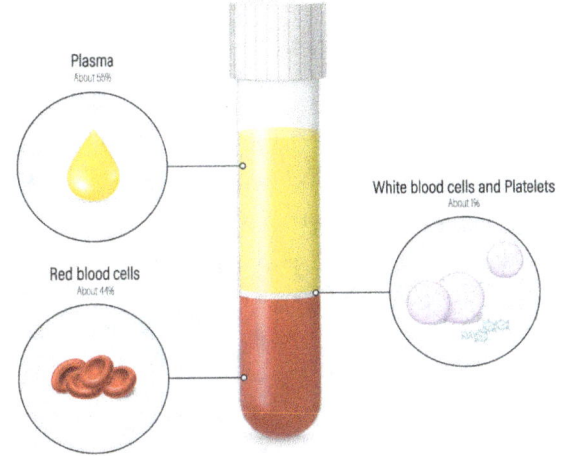

Red blood cells

Red blood cells make up about **40-45% of the volume of blood**. Their function is to carry oxygen from the lungs to the rest of the body.

Adaptations that help them transport as much oxygen as possible:
- Biconcave disc shape increases surface area to absorb more oxygen.
- No nucleus, so more space is available to carry haemoglobin.

Haemoglobin is a protein containing iron that easily binds with oxygen.
- Each haemoglobin molecule binds with 4 oxygen molecules.
- When haemoglobin binds with oxygen it becomes **oxyhaemoglobin**.

Plasma

Plasma makes up about **55% of the volume of blood**. Its function is to transport substances such as:
- Nutrients.
- Waste products like urea.
- Hormones.
- Plasma proteins (e.g. antibodies and clotting factors).

Plasma makes the blood thinner (less viscous) so it can flow more easily through the blood vessels. If there is an increase in plasma proteins, blood viscosity increases which slows the flow of blood.

Platelets

Platelets make up **less than 1% of the volume of blood**. Their function is to help blood clot.

The process of blood clotting is:
- The platelets are activated and become spiky.
- Proteins called blood clotting factors are activated and start a chain reaction to produce an insoluble protein called **fibrin**.
- Fibrin creates a tangled web around the spiky platelets. Together they form the clot.

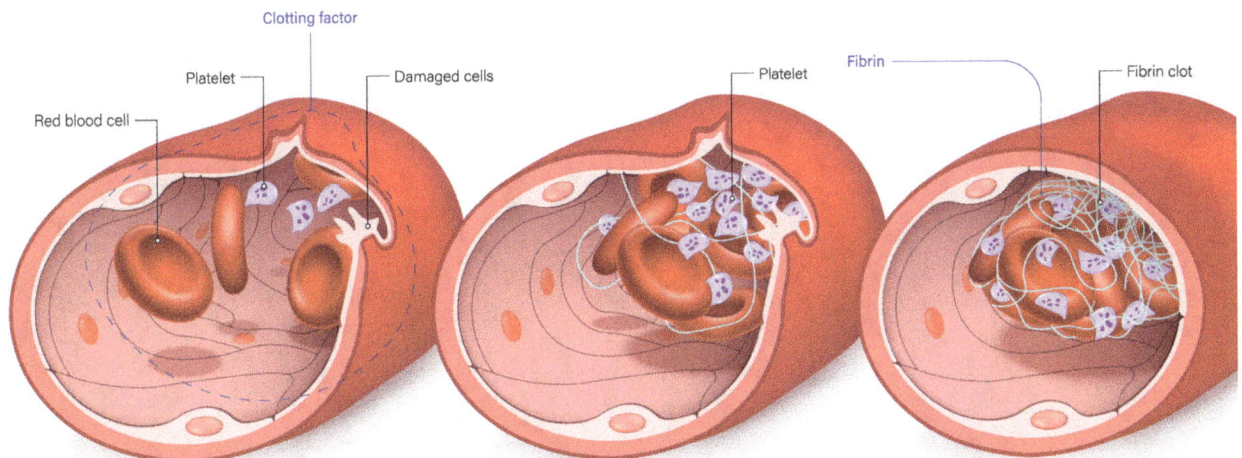

1.2 The heart

Structure of the heart

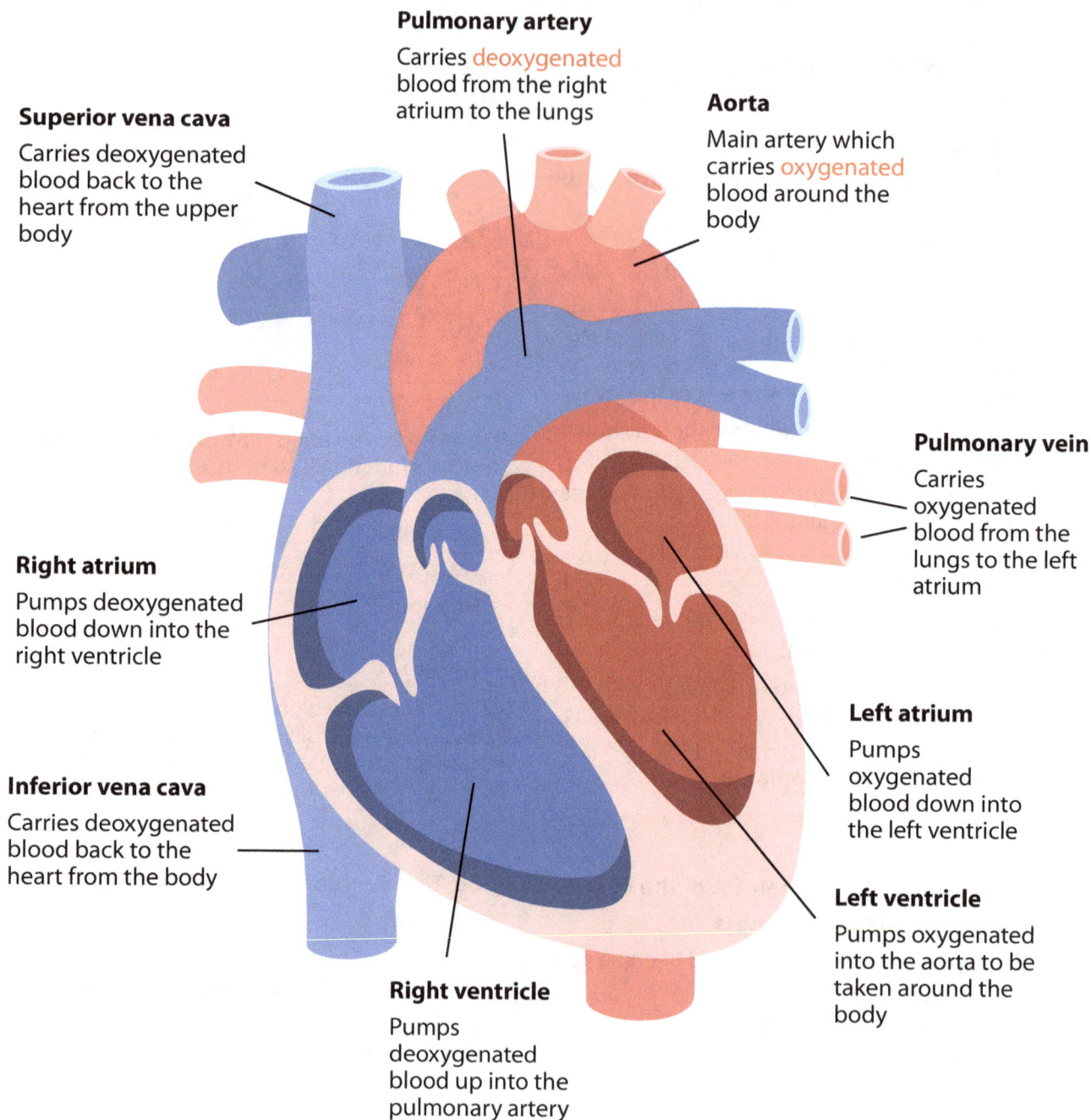

Valves

Semi-lunar pulmonary valve
At the bottom of the pulmonary artery. Stops blood flowing back into the right ventricle

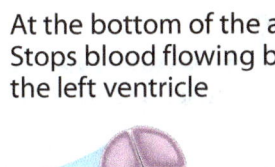

Semi-lunar aortic valve
At the bottom of the aorta. Stops blood flowing back into the left ventricle

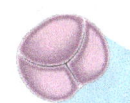

Cardiac tissue
Type of muscle tissue that the heart walls are made of

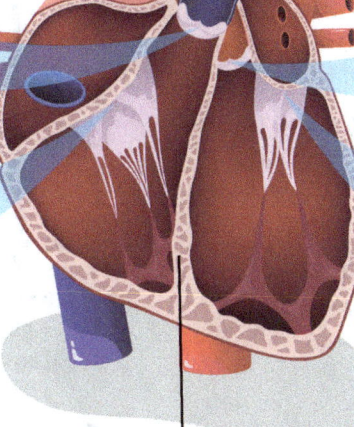

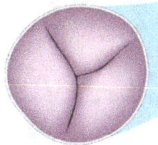

Tricuspid valve
Between the right atrium and right ventricle. Prevents backflow of blood back into atrium

Septum
Wall that separates the left and right sides of the heart

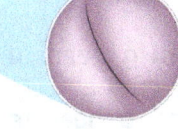

Bicuspid valve
Between the left atrium and left ventricle. Prevents backflow of blood back into atrium

Other structures

- The **septum** separates the left and right sides of the heart.
- **Cardiac tissue** is the tissue that makes up the walls of the heart. It is made of cardiac muscle, which contracts to make the heart pump.
- **Coronary arteries** extend from the base of the aorta around the outside of the heart to supply the heart walls with oxygen and nutrients.

The flow of blood through the heart

The flow of blood through the heart is as follows:

- 1: Deoxygenated blood passes from both **vena cava veins** into the **right atrium**.
- 2: Deoxygenated blood is pumped through the **tricuspid valve** into the **right ventricle.**
- 3: Deoxygenated blood is pumped through the **semi-lunar pulmonary valve** into the **pulmonary artery** and travels to the lungs to pick up oxygen.
- 4: Oxygenated blood returns to the **left atrium** via the **pulmonary veins**.
- 5: Oxygenated blood is pumped from the **left atrium**, through the **bicuspid valve**, into the **left ventricle**.
- 6: Oxygenated blood is pumped through the **semi-lunar aortic** valve into the **aorta**, to be then transported around the body.

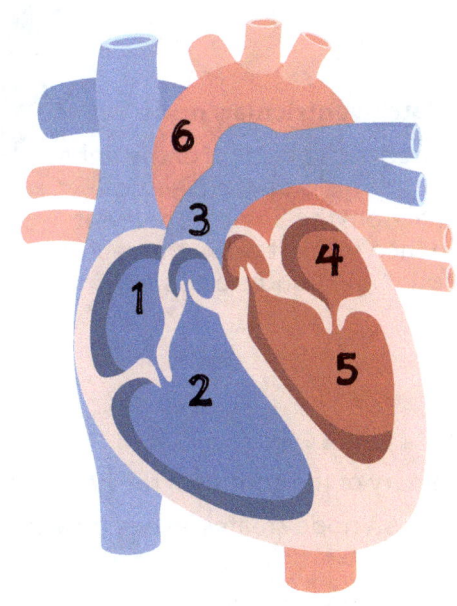

1: Cardiovascular system

Blood pressure

Blood pressure is the force of the blood against the blood vessel walls.

- During the **systolic phase** of the heartbeat, the heart muscles are contracting. **Systolic pressure** is high.
- During the **diastolic phase** of the heartbeat, the heart muscles relax. **Diastolic pressure** is lower.
- The ideal range of blood pressure is between 90/60 mmHg and 120/80 mmHg.
  » Low blood pressure is below 90/90 mmHg.
  » High blood pressure is above 120/80 mmHg.

mmHg means 'millimetres of mercury' and is the unit of pressure used to measure blood pressure.

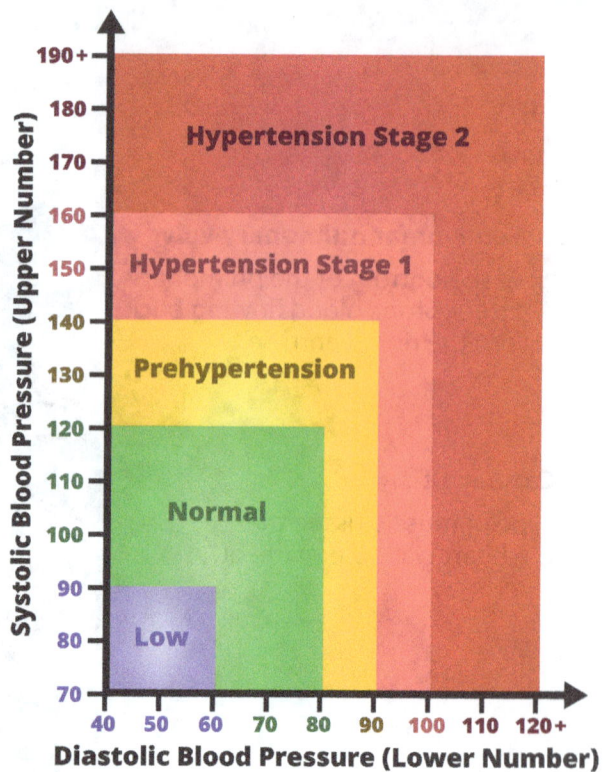

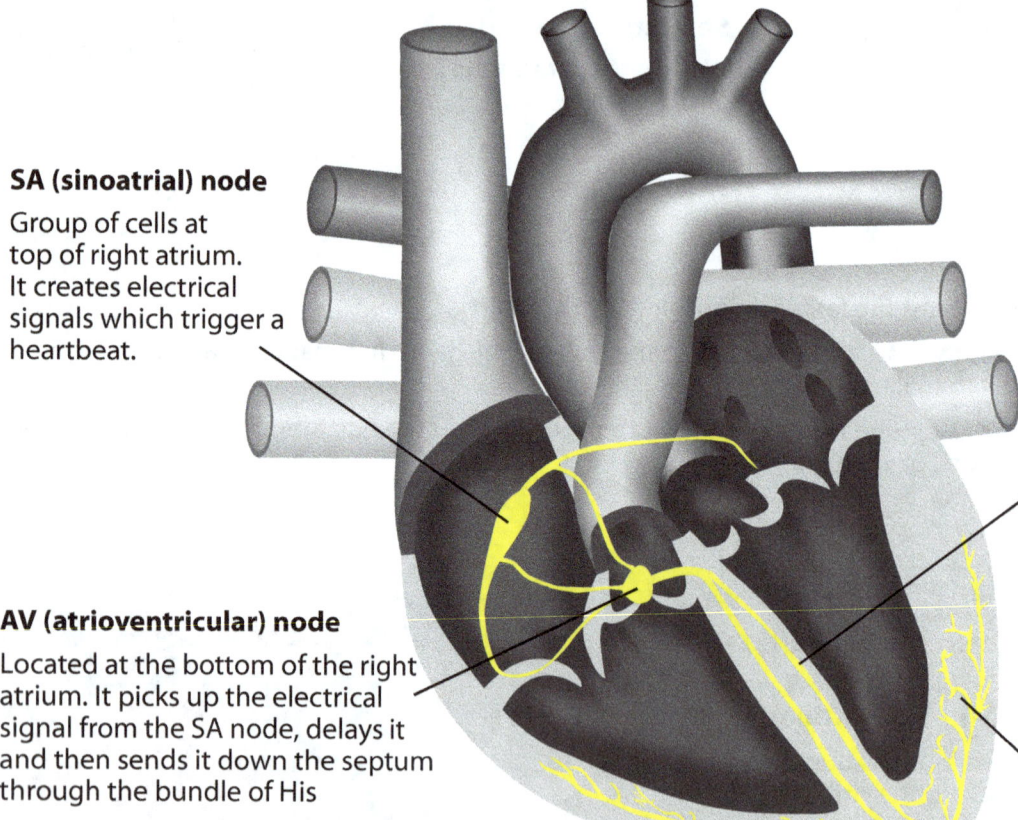

SA (sinoatrial) node
Group of cells at top of right atrium. It creates electrical signals which trigger a heartbeat.

AV (atrioventricular) node
Located at the bottom of the right atrium. It picks up the electrical signal from the SA node, delays it and then sends it down the septum through the bundle of His

Bundle of His
Runs down the septum to the apex of the heart.
It carries the electrical signal from the atria down to the bottom of the ventricles to the Purkinje fibres

Purkinje (Purkyne) fibres
Run throughout the walls of the ventricles from the bottom up. They cause the ventricles to contract.

Electrical activity of the heart

Summary of the control of the heartbeat:

- The SA node creates an electrical impulse that travels through the atria walls, causing them to contract.
- The AV node picks up the signal and delays it, then sends the signal to the Bundle of His.
- Electrical signals pass down the septum of the ventricles to the bottom (apex) of the heart through the Bundle of His.
- Electrical signals pass from the Bundle of His into the Purkinje fibres, causing the ventricles to contract.

Electrocardiogram (ECG) trace

An ECG trace is used by the medical profession to check for problems with the heartbeat.

- **P wave** – Shows electrical impulse in the SA node. Represents atria contracting.
- **QRS wave** – Shows electrical signals from the AV node, Bundle of His and Purkinje fibres. It represents the contraction of the ventricles.
- **T wave** – Shows the repolarisation of the ventricles (when they prepare for the next contraction). Represents relaxation of the ventricles.

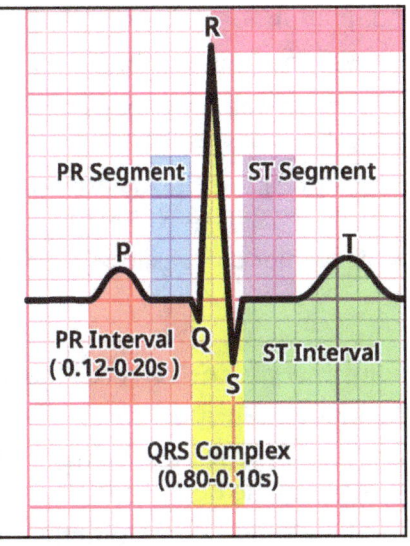

Some abnormal ECG traces are as follows:

- **Tachycardia** – heartbeat over 100 bpm. The PQRST waves are closer together.
- **Bradycardia** – slow heartbeat of less than 60 bpm. PQRST waves will be further apart.
- **Atrial fibrillation** – atria are not contracting properly. It will be difficult to see the P wave.
- **Ventricular fibrillation** – ventricles are not contracting properly. No obvious PQRST pattern. This is an emergency.

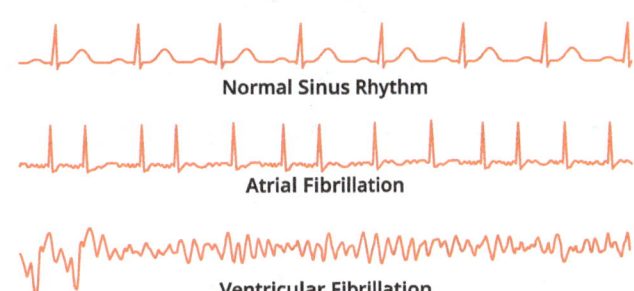

1.3 Blood vessels

Arteries

Arteries **carry blood away** from the heart.

Adaptations include:

- Thick muscular walls to withstand high blood pressure.
- Elastic walls in order to push blood further along the artery and return the artery to normal size after a heartbeat.
- Narrow lumen to maintain high blood pressure, helping blood pass quickly through the arteries.

Capillaries

The function of capillaries is to **exchange substances with the tissues** of the body:

- Oxygen passes from the bloodstream into the tissues (apart from in the lungs).
- Nutrients, such as glucose, fats and amino acids, pass from the bloodstream into the tissues.
- Hormones pass from the bloodstream into the tissues where they are meant to act.
- Hormones also enter bloodstream from the tissues where they are produced (e.g. the pancreas)..
- Waste products, such as urea, pass from the tissues into the bloodstream.
- Carbon dioxide passes from the tissues into the bloodstream.

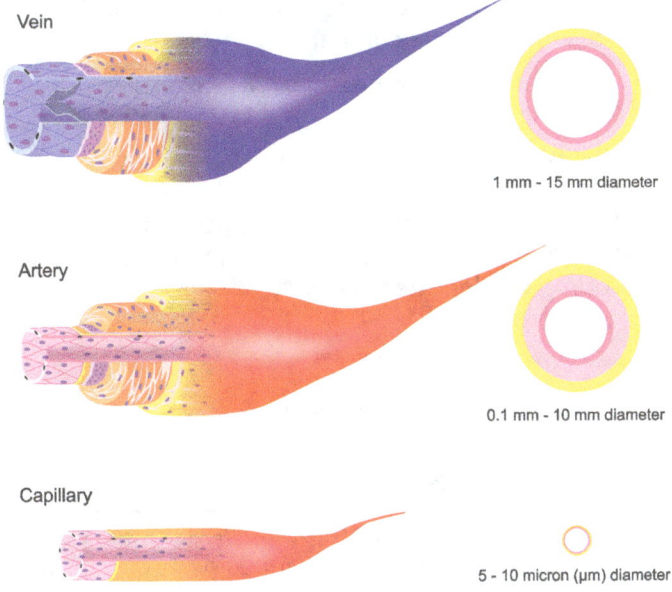

Adaptations of the capillaries:

- Walls are one cell thick, so substances have less far to travel to get into or out of the blood.
- Porous wall (small gaps between cells that make up the capillary walls) so substances can get into and out of the capillary easily.
- Narrow lumen slows down blood flow and forces red blood cells to squeeze close to the walls, so that oxygen can leave more easily.
- Slow blood flow allows substances time to pass into and out of the blood.

Veins

Veins **carry blood towards** the heart.

Adaptations include:

- Wide lumen to reduce friction between blood and the walls and allows more blood to be carried back to the heart.
- Semi-lunar valves along the length of the veins prevent blood from flowing in the wrong direction so it can get back to the heart.

1.4 Conditions of the cardiovascular system

Angina

People with **angina** get a pain in the chest, particularly after they have been doing some activity. It is due to the narrowing of the coronary artery that supplies the heart muscle, meaning less blood reaches the heart muscle.

Causes

- **Atheroma** – a build-up of fatty plaque under the lining of the coronary artery.
- This causes a **narrowing of the coronary arteries**.

When blood cannot get through the narrowed arteries, the heart muscle does not get enough oxygen and nutrients and cannot pump properly. This is more noticeable when the heart is trying to pump harder due to activity.

Symptoms

- Tight chest.
- Chest pains that spread to the arms, neck and jaw.
- Breathlessness as not enough oxygen is getting to the heart muscle, so you breathe quicker to get more oxygen.

NORMAL FUNCTIONS

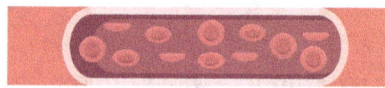

CHOLESTEROL PLAQUE FORMATION

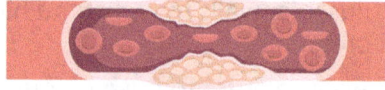

COMPLETE BLOCKAGE

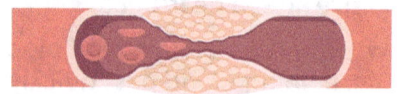

Diagnosis and monitoring

	Description	When it is used	Results
ECG	Electrocardiogram – electrodes are attached to various parts of the body. It detects the electrical activity of the heart and produces an ECG trace.	It will only show differences in an ECG trace if taken during an angina attack.	The T wave becomes flattened or even inverted.
Angiogram	A dye is injected into the bloodstream and then an X-ray is taken.	It can be used to find blocked coronary arteries during diagnosis. It can be used to monitor whether new arteries become blocked.	Blocked arteries become visible.

	Description	When it is used	Results
Blood tests	Blood tests are taken to look for chemicals that show the blood vessels are damaged.	Used if angina is suspected. Can also be used to detect high fat and cholesterol levels to see if people are at risk of developing the disease.	Cannot diagnose the condition by itself.

Treatments

Surgical	Non-surgical
Angioplasty	Nitrolingual pump
Coronary bypass	Anticoagulants

Angioplasty

- A balloon is used to open the blocked coronary artery.
- A stent (wire mesh) is then inserted to keep it open.
- Both balloon and stent are inserted through a tube called a catheter, which is threaded through the cardiovascular system from the wrist or groin.

Benefits	Limitations
Symptoms are relieved immediately.	There is a risk of infection at the catheter insertion point.
Reduces the risk of heart attacks	The stent can cause more plaque to build up.

Coronary bypass

A blood vessel from elsewhere in the body is used to bypass the blocked section of coronary artery.

Benefits	Limitations
Symptoms improved immediately.	Major surgery increases the risk of bleeding, blood clot formation and infection.
Risk of heart attack reduced.	The surgery can cause irregular heartbeats (arrhythmia).
The life of the individual is prolonged.	Increased risk of developing kidney and breathing difficulties.

Angioplasty

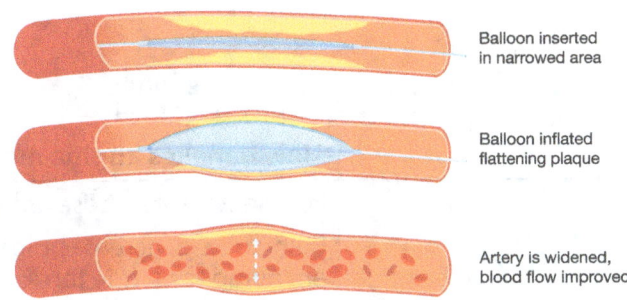

Balloon inserted in narrowed area

Balloon inflated flattening plaque

Artery is widened, blood flow improved

Nitrolingual pump

Nitrolingual pumps are used during an angina attack to ease the symptoms. The medication is sprayed under the tongue. It causes the blood vessels to dilate (get wider) so blood can flow more easily.

Benefits	Limitations
Relief from pain is almost immediate.	It does not treat the blockages caused by atheroma.
It can be used before physical activity to prevent angina pain.	Side effects include headaches and dizziness.
It is easy and convenient to carry.	Only three doses can be given in 15 minutes, so it may not be enough for some people.
It does not involve swallowing tablets, which is difficult for some people.	It is not suitable for people with low blood pressure as it lowers pressure.

Anticoagulant

Anticoagulant medication prevents the formation of blood clots, preventing the condition from getting worse. They tend to be used to lower the risk of heart attacks.

Benefits	Limitations
Reduces the risk of heart attacks and **ischaemic strokes** (see later).	It does not remove blood clots that have already formed.
It is useful after surgery to prevent blood clots from forming.	Blood may not be able to clot when it needs to, so it can lead to excessive bleeding.
They improve blood flow in general, so other organs benefit.	Some foods need to be avoided, such as grapefruit, cranberries, kale, egg yolks and certain cheeses.

Factors that make angina more likely

Factor	How it makes angina more likely
Obesity	People who are obese are more likely to have a high-fat diet.
	Being obese increases blood pressure which damages blood vessels and encourages plaque formation.
	More blood needs to be pumped around the body, increasing strain on the heart.
High-fat or high-salt diet	Fat in the diet encourages plaque and atheroma formation.
	Salt increases blood pressure which damages blood vessels.
Smoking	Chemicals in cigarette smoke damage blood vessels.
	Smoking makes it harder for the blood to carry oxygen, putting strain on the heart.
	Smoking increases heart rate and blood pressure.
Diabetes	High blood sugar levels due to diabetes damage blood vessels.
	Inflammation increases with diabetes and encourages plaque formation.
	Blood clots more easily.
Stress	Increases blood pressure.
	Stress may make a person more likely to eat unhealthy food and smoke.

Control and prevention

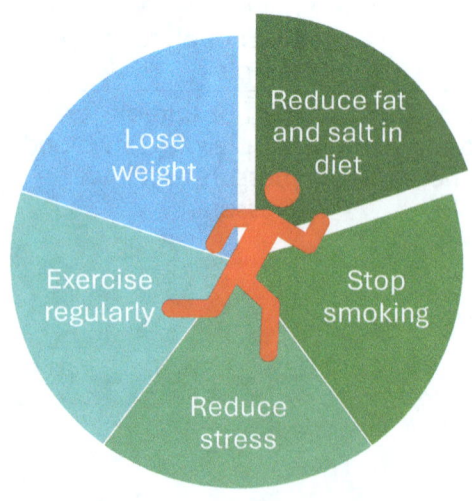

- Reducing fat discourages plaque formation.
- Reducing salt reduces blood pressure.
- Stopping smoking reduces harmful chemicals and increases the blood's ability to carry oxygen.
- Reducing stress reduces blood pressure and discourages poor diet.
- Exercising regularly improves condition of the heart, lowers blood pressure, reduces stress and discourages plaque formation.
- Losing weight discourages plaque formation and reduces strain on the heart.

Impact of angina on the individual

Physical	Intellectual
- Pain in the chest - Feeling tired - Breathlessness	- Difficulty focusing - Difficulty making decisions
Emotional	**Social**
- Anxiety about heart attacks - Difficult changes in lifestyle needed - Feeling that they are to blame - Low self-esteem	- Difficulty going out and socialising - Social withdrawal and isolation - May become dependent on other people - Possible conflict with friends and family due to dependency

Deep vein thrombosis (DVT)

A thrombosis is a blood clot. Deep vein thrombosis is when a blood clot forms in veins that lie deep in the body.

Causes

- Blood clots forming in deep veins – leading to pain and swelling in the area.
- Restricted blood flow due to blockages.
- Most common in legs and pelvis.
- Clots can break off and travel to the lungs, causing a **pulmonary embolism**.

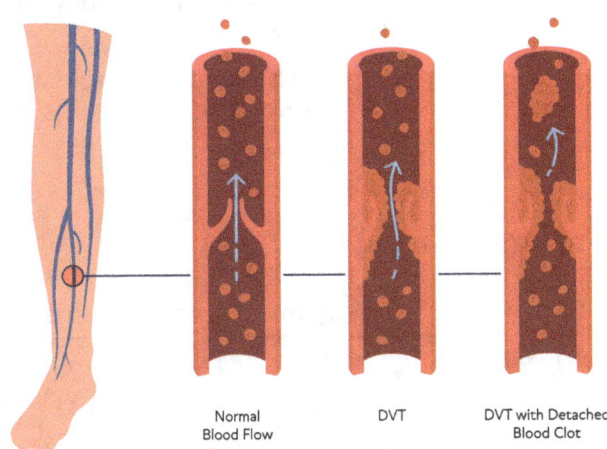

Normal Blood Flow   DVT   DVT with Detached Blood Clot

Pulmonary embolism

Where an artery in the lungs becomes blocked. This damages lung tissue

Signs and symptoms

- Pain (such as in the leg where the blocked vessel is).
- Swelling of area.
- Redness of the skin where the blockage is.

Diagnosis and monitoring

Method	Details	Use in diagnosis	Use in monitoring
Ultrasound scan	High-frequency sound waves are used to make a picture of the scanned area.	Can detect blockages in veins.	Can check if the thrombosis is getting smaller after treatment. Checks that no new clots are forming.
Venography	Special dye is injected into the blood. Blood clots can now show up on an X-ray.	Used to locate blockage for diagnosis and treatment.	Used to see if treatment is working.

Treatments

- **Anticoagulant medicine** prevents further clots from forming.
- **Thrombolytics** break down clots that have already formed.
- **Thrombectomy** removes the blood clot using a suction tube inserted into the affected vein.
- **Filters** prevent clots from travelling to the lungs if they break away. Filters are usually placed in the inferior vena cava.

	Advantages	Disadvantages
Anticoagulant medicine	• Reduces risk of heart attacks, strokes and pulmonary embolisms • Prevents new clots • Improves blood flow	• Does not remove existing clots • Can lead to excessive bleeding • Do not work with some food, such as grapefruit
Thrombolytics	• Removes clots that have already formed • Reduces the risk of heart attacks, strokes and pulmonary embolisms	• Can lead to excessive bleeding • Can increase the risk of a haemorrhagic stroke • Does not prevent new clots from forming
Thrombectomy	• Relieves symptoms straight away • Reduces the risk of heart attacks, strokes and pulmonary embolism	• Risk of local infection at site of cut to blood vessel • Can damage blood vessels
Filters	• Reduce the risk of pulmonary embolism • Can be used by people who cannot take anticoagulants • Can be removed	• Do not prevent blood clots from forming • Blood clots can form at the site of the filter • Can be difficult to remove

Factors making DVT more likely

Factor	Why this increases the risk
Age 60+	• Veins are less elastic, and clots form more easily • People often move less when older • Older people may do less exercise • They are more likely to have developed diseases that increase the risk of blood clots
Being overweight	• Clots are more likely to form if you are overweight • Some overweight people exercise less • It is harder for blood to get back to the heart, so it is more likely to clot • Blood clots more easily when you are overweight
Smoking	• Chemicals in cigarette smoke encourage clotting • Smoking damages the blood vessels, making clots more likely • Smoking affects blood circulation, making it harder for blood to return to the heart
Contraceptive medication	• The oestrogen pill increases the risk of DVT • Oestrogen makes blood clot more easily • The effect of oestrogen can be made worse if the person has genetic factors as well
Hormone replacement therapy (HRT)	• HRT increases oestrogen levels in the body • Oestrogen makes the blood clot more easily
Previous DVT	• The things that caused the previous DVT are still likely to be there • They are more likely to have already damaged blood vessels
Flying and restricted movement	• Lack of movement makes it harder for blood to get back to the heart as it relies on leg muscles contracting • Lack of movement makes blood clot more easily • Low air pressure in aeroplanes thickens the blood, making it clot more easily

Control and prevention

- **Compression stockings** squeeze the veins in the legs, helping blood flow and preventing clots.
- **Regular movement** causes the leg muscles to squeeze the veins in the legs to reduce blood clot risk.
- **Hydration** makes blood flow more easily, so it is less likely to clot. Many older people do not drink enough water.
- **Lifestyle changes** lessen some of the risk factors such as not moving enough, smoking, fatty or salty diet and not drinking enough.

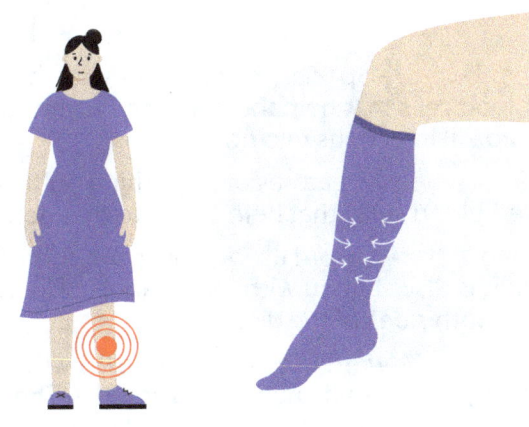

Impact of DVT on the individual

Physical	Intellectual
• Pain • Damage to the area affected • Less likely to exercise due to discomfort • A clot can break away and cause a pulmonary embolism	• May need to miss education or work, affecting intellectual development • Less likely to carry out intellectually stimulating activities
Emotional	**Social**
• Anxiety about the consequences of the condition • Depression caused by the impact of the condition • Stress due to treatment and control measures	• Difficulty going out and socialising • Social withdrawal and isolation • May become dependent on other people • Possible conflict with friends and family due to dependency

Study Tips!

- It is important that you are able to explain how each component of blood is **adapted** to carry out its function.
- Remember that the right-hand side of the heart on a diagram is on your left-hand side.
- Remember that in a diagram of the heart, red represents oxygenated blood and blue represents deoxygenated blood.
- It is important to know which way blood flows through the heart – which chambers and vessels the blood goes through and in which order.
- You need to know when each valve opens and closes.
- Most biological names should be written with a small first letter unless at the beginning of a sentence. However, Purkinje and His are exceptions and must be capitalised as they were named after people.
- You can think of 'electrical impulse' and 'electrical signals' as being very similar to nerve impulses but these signals travel through muscle cells rather than neurones.
- You need to know what is happening at each stage of a PQRST trace (or ECG trace) and what a normal and abnormal trace might look like.
- You need to be able to explain how the structure of each type of blood vessel helps it to do its specific job.
- You may need to look at pictures of angiograms and decide whether blood vessels are blocked.
- You will need to understand advantages and disadvantages of different treatments so that you can justify why a particular treatment may be better for a particular person.

Important terms!

Antibodies – Special proteins produced by white blood cells that help the immune system to find and kill infectious microorganisms.

Adaptations – features of something (in this case red blood cells) that help them do their job.

Biconcave – A word used to describe something that is disc-shaped with indentations (like caves) on both sides of the disc.

Viscous – A word used to describe how thick and sticky versus thin and runny a liquid is. The more viscous a liquid is, the thicker and stickier it is.

Blood clotting factor - Proteins that circulate in the bloodstream as part of the plasma. They control clotting of the blood. There are many different types, all of which are necessary for the blood to clot.

Deoxygenated - Blood that has given up its oxygen to cells, so it is no longer carrying oxygen. It is shown in blue on diagrams of the heart and circulatory system.

Oxygenated – Blood that is carrying oxygen within the red blood cells. It is shown in red on diagrams of the heart and circulatory system.

mmHg – A shortened version of "millimetres of mercury". It is the unit of pressure used for blood pressure.

Apex - The pointed lower end of the heart.

Repolarisation - The process of the neurone returning to its resting state after a nerve impulse. When it has repolarised it is ready to fire again.

Lumen - The inside space of a tube e.g. a blood vessel or the intestines.

Porous – Something that has tiny gaps or spaces in its wall that let some gases or liquids pass through.

Plaque - A sticky build-up of substances such as fat, cholesterol and calcium inside the walls of blood vessels.

Inverted – Upside down or the wrong way up. In the case of an ECG trace, the graph would show a trough instead of a peak.

Stent - A short mesh tube that can be placed into a blood vessel to prevent the walls from narrowing. They are often opened up when in the correct position by using a balloon.

Catheter – A thin, flexible tube which can be inserted into the body. The catheters described in this section are inserted into veins in the cardiovascular system.

Arrhythmia - Any irregularity in the pattern of heartbeats. Examples include beating too quickly or too slowly.

Anticoagulant – A medicine which makes it harder for the blood to clot.

Haemorrhagic stroke – A stroke caused by a bleed into the brain (in contrast to an ischaemic stroke, which is caused by a blood clot in the brain.)

Recap Questions

1. What percentage of blood is made up of white blood cells?
2. What is the role of plasma?
3. What adaptations do red blood cells have to allow them to carry more oxygen?
4. What is fibrin?
5. Name the four chambers of the heart.
6. What is the ideal range for blood pressure readings?
7. What are three differences between veins and arteries.
8. What are two symptoms of angina?
9. Name a non-surgical treatment for angina.
10. Why is a smoker more likely to develop angina than a non-smoker?
11. What is deep vein thrombosis (DVT)?
12. How can venography diagnose DVT?
13. What are the physical impacts of DVT?
14. Name one lifestyle change an individual can make to control DVT.

Revision Quiz

1. a) Name all of the person-centred values of care.

   b) Explain why you think the person-centred values of care are important.
2. Give an example of a neurological disorder.
3. Where in the body is the humerus?
4. How can an eye test help diagnose type 2 diabetes?
5. What role does obesity play in the development of gallstones?
6. What is the role of the trachea?
7. What is a diffusion gradient?
8. Name one symptom of carpal tunnel syndrome.
9. What is a peak flow meter and how is it used to manage asthma?
10. Describe an emotional impact of gallstones on an individual.
11. Which type of joint allows the greatest range of movement?
12. What is the function of tissue fluid during absorption?
13. What dietary changes can someone make to reduce their risk of ischaemic strokes?
14. What features of osteoarthritis might be visible in an X-ray?
15. What is a peripheral nerve?
16. What is FSH?

Assessment practice

1. Identify two ways in which white blood cells protect against infection. (2)
2. What is the function of red blood cells? (1)

   A to fight disease

   B to carry oxygen

   C to help blood clot

   D to carry nutrients
3. Identify the parts of the heart in the diagram below. (4)

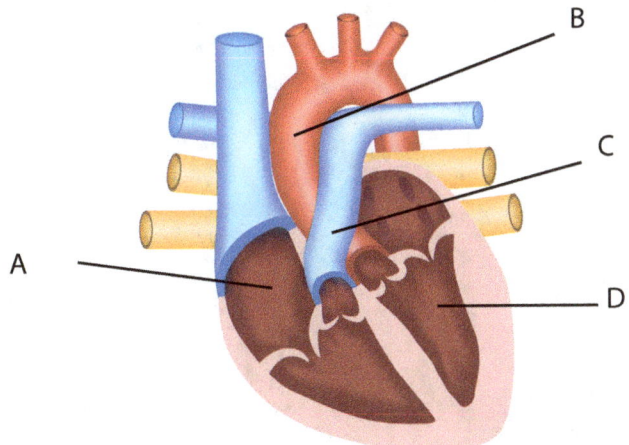

4. State the name of the valve that lies between the left atrium and the left ventricle. (1)

5. Fill in the gaps: The _____ valves are at the base of the arteries and prevent blood flowing back to the heart. The _____ valve is the one that is at the base of the aorta. (2)

6. What is the name of the type of blood pressure caused when the heart is contracting? (1)

7. State what the heart muscle is doing during the diastolic phase. (1)

8. Fill in the gaps: The _____ node is located at the top right of the right atrium and the _____ node is at the base of the right atrium. (2)

9. What does the P wave represent in an ECG trace? (1)

10. Fill in the gaps: Arteries carry _____ blood _____ from the heart and _____ organs. (2)

11. Under which blood pressure do the muscles in the artery walls contract? (1)

12. Which statement is correct about veins? (1)

    A Veins always carry deoxygenated blood
    B Veins carry blood towards organs
    C Veins carry blood towards the heart

13. What is the name of the special type of X-ray which can show whether blood vessels in the heart are blocked when diagnosing angina? (1)

14. State two lifestyle changes that will help control or prevent angina. (2)

15. State the name of the type of medicine that makes it harder for blood to clot that is used in the treatment of DVT. (1)

16. What components of the contraceptive pill and HRT makes DVT more likely to develop? (2)

17. Explain how white blood cells protect the body against infection (3)

18. Explain how the valves ensure blood flows in the correct direction (4)

19. Explain why a GP may be concerned about an individual with a blood pressure of 140/90? (2)

20. Explain what happens during the systolic and diastolic phases of the heartbeat. (3)

21. Explain how blood in veins can flow back to the heart despite low pressure. (3)

22. Analyse the effects of angina on an individual. (6)

23. Describe the use of ultrasound scans to diagnose DVT. (4)

24. Discuss the treatments available for DVT. (9)

2: Respiratory system

2.1 Structure and function of the respiratory system

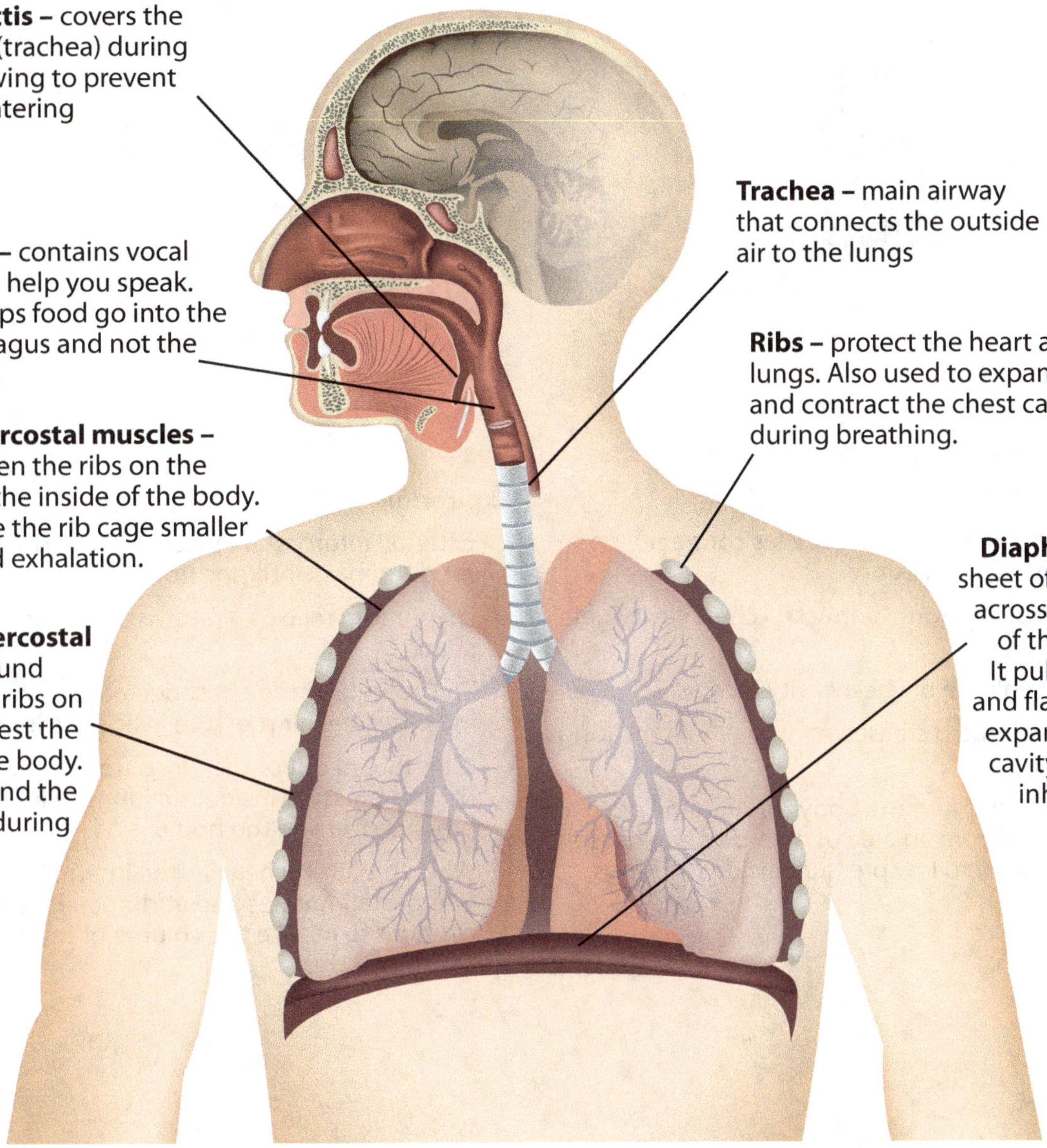

Epiglottis – covers the airway (trachea) during swallowing to prevent food entering

Larynx – contains vocal cords to help you speak. Also helps food go into the oesophagus and not the trachea.

Internal intercostal muscles – found between the ribs on the side nearest the inside of the body. Used to make the rib cage smaller during forced exhalation.

External intercostal muscles – found between the ribs on the side nearest the outside of the body. Used to expand the chest cavity during inhaling.

Trachea – main airway that connects the outside air to the lungs

Ribs – protect the heart and lungs. Also used to expand and contract the chest cavity during breathing.

Diaphragm – sheet of muscle across bottom of the lungs. It pulls down and flattens to expand chest cavity during inhalation.

Pleural membrane – double layer of membrane which surrounds the lungs and covers the inside wall of the chest cavity. Makes sure the lungs expand when the chest expands so that we can breathe.

Pleural fluid – fluid between the two layers of the pleural membrane. It allows the two membrane to slide past each other but prevents them being pulled apart.

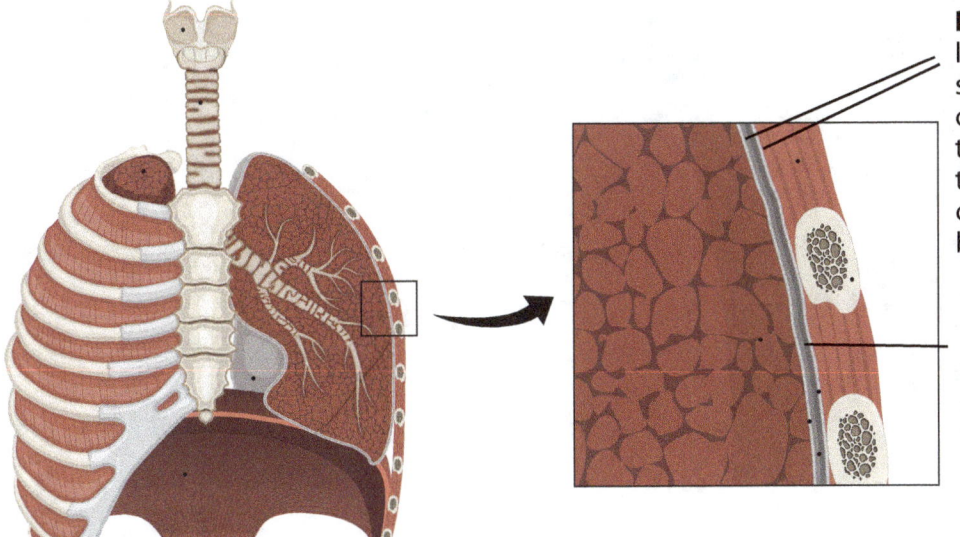

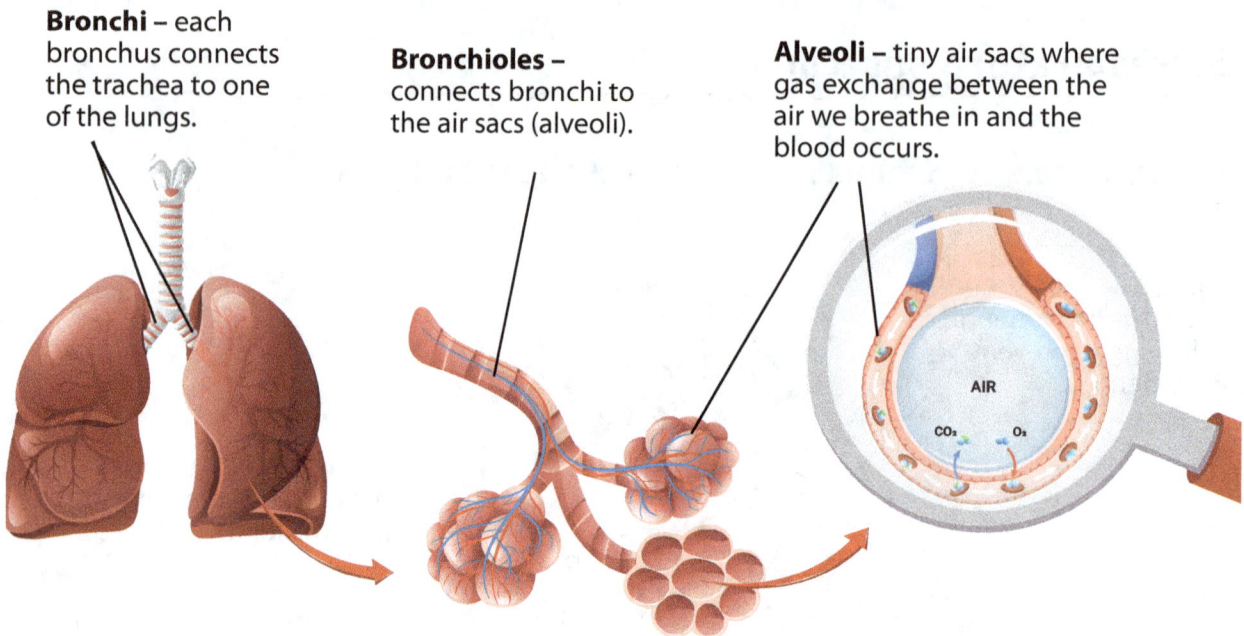

Bronchi – each bronchus connects the trachea to one of the lungs.

Bronchioles – connects bronchi to the air sacs (alveoli).

Alveoli – tiny air sacs where gas exchange between the air we breathe in and the blood occurs.

2.2 Mechanics of breathing

Inspiration
- External intercostal muscles contract – ribs move up and out.
- The diaphragm contracts – chest cavity gets bigger.
- The volume of chest cavity increases.
- As volume increases, air pressure in the lungs decreases.
- Air rushes into the body through the nose and mouth from an area of high pressure outside the body to low pressure inside the lungs.

Expiration
- External intercostal muscles relax – ribs rebound back into position.
- Diaphragm relaxes – returns to its domed shape.
- The volume of the chest decreases, which increases the air pressure inside the lungs.
- Air is forced out of the lungs from an area of high pressure inside the lungs to lower pressure outside the body.
- When breathing heavily, the internal intercostal muscles and abdominal muscles contract to reduce the volume of the chest cavity quicker.

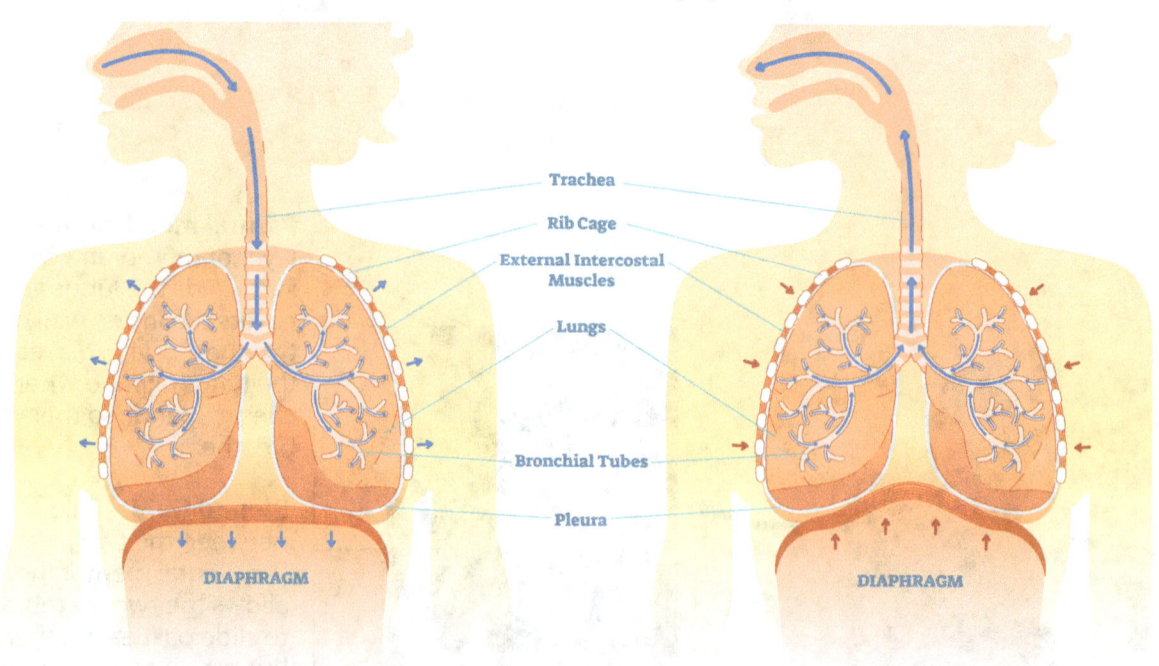

Inspiration

Expiration

2.3 Gaseous exchange

- Both oxygen and carbon dioxide diffuse across the alveoli wall from an area of high concentration to an area of low concentration.
- Oxygen diffuses from the alveoli into the blood.
- Carbon dioxide diffuses from the blood into the alveoli.

Haemoglobin

- **Haemoglobin** is a protein combined with iron and is carried in red blood cells.
  » Four oxygen molecules can combine with each haemoglobin molecule.
  » Haemoglobin is used to carry oxygen in the blood to where it is needed.

Alveoli

- Alveoli are where **gas exchange** takes place.
- The walls are very thin and made of epithelial tissue.
- Because they are thin, oxygen and carbon dioxide do not have far to travel.

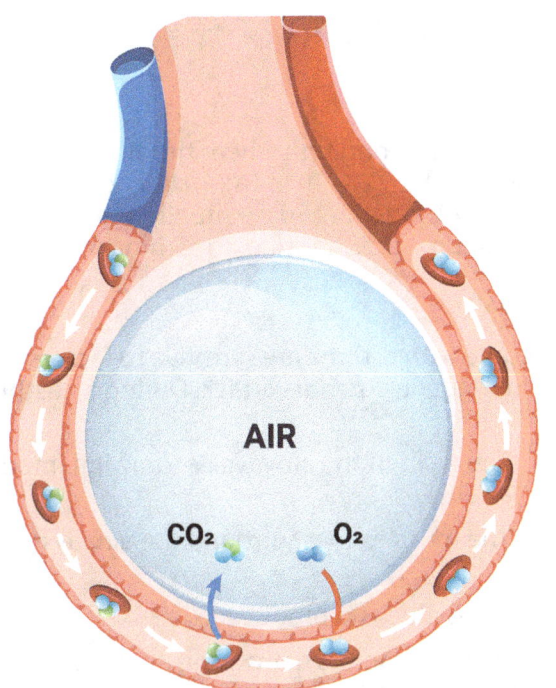

Diffusion gradient

A **diffusion gradient** exists where there is a difference in concentrations of a gas (or liquid) in different areas.

» Gases diffuse from an area of high concentration to an area of low concentration.
» The concentration of oxygen is high in the alveoli and low in the blood – so oxygen diffuses from alveoli to blood.
» The concentration of carbon dioxide is low in the alveoli but high in the blood – so carbon dioxide diffuses from blood to alveoli.

2.4 Cellular respiration

Aerobic respiration uses glucose and oxygen to generate energy for the body. It takes place in the cells, mostly in structures within the cell (organelles) called mitochondria.

Oxygen + Glucose → Energy + Water + Carbon Dioxide

Anaerobic respiration gets energy out of glucose but does not need oxygen. It takes place in the cytoplasm of cells (not in mitochondria).

Glucose → Energy + Lactic Acid

Both forms of respiration make a molecule called ATP (adenosine triphosphate). ATP can provide energy quickly for the cell.

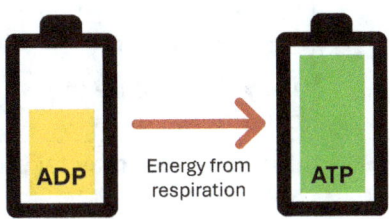

Aerobic respiration creates many more molecules of ATP than anaerobic respiration

2.5 Conditions of the respiratory system

Asthma

Asthma is a condition where the airways narrow due to *inflammation* of the walls and excess mucus production. Some situations make the condition worse, causing an asthma attack.

Causes

People with asthma are sensitive to factors that can trigger an asthma attack. During an asthma attack:

- The walls of the airways become inflamed and swell.
- The muscles that surround the airways *constrict*.
- More mucus is produced.

normal airway   asthmatic airway   during attack

These three factors narrow the airways, so it is harder to breathe in and out. This means that gaseous exchange is reduced, so less oxygen gets into the bloodstream.

Signs and symptoms

- Wheezing.
- Coughing.
- Tight chest.
- Breathlessness.

Diagnosis and monitoring

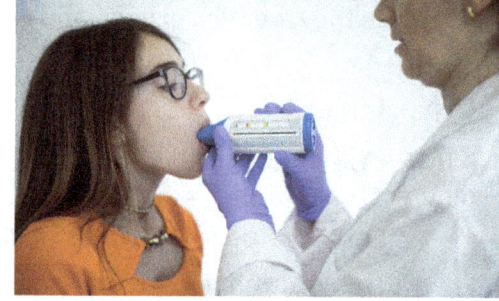

Peak flow meter

Peak flow meters measure how fast air can be blown out. The patient needs to blow through the device as hard as possible. The reading will depend on age, sex and height. Low readings indicate problems with the lungs, which may be asthma.

Peak flow meters are also used for monitoring whether the asthma is being managed well. If readings are lower than normal, stronger medication may be needed.

A **spirometer** is used with a computer and can show different readings:

- How much a person can breathe out have taking a deep breath (forced vital capacity).
- How forcefully a person can breathe out (forced expiratory volume in one second).
- The ratio between the first two readings.

If the readings improve after the patient has been given a drug to open the airways, the condition is likely to be asthma rather than other lung conditions.

Spirometers can also be used to check treatments are working.

Treatments

Treatment	Details	Advantages	Disadvantages
Reliever inhaler	• Used when symptoms are worse. • A dose is breathed in from the device. • The medication causes the airways to *dilate* (widen).	Relieves symptoms during an asthma attack. Easy to carry.	Can cause a dry mouth and can make you feel sick. Become less effective if used too much. They do not cure the condition.
Preventer inhaler	• Taken daily. • Reduces sensitivity to triggers.	Prevents asthma attacks. Reduces the number of asthma attacks.	Improvement may take a few weeks. Side effects include sore throat and hoarse voice.

Treatment	Details	Advantages	Disadvantages
Steroidal tablets	• Prescribed during severe asthma attacks or for chest infections. • Reduces inflammation of the airways.	They can be quick acting. They prevent asthma attacks and can save lives.	Long term use can cause weight gain. Can cause high blood pressure, weaker bones and mood changes.
Nebuliser	• Medication is broken down into a mist which is breathed in through a face mask for about 20 minutes. • It relaxes the muscles around the airways making them wider.	They are easy to use. They can give higher doses of medication. Very useful for more severe asthma attacks.	They need to be plugged in so cannot be used everywhere. They take longer to work. The machine will need to be cleaned and maintained.

Factors making asthma more likely

- **Family history** makes asthma more likely but not certain
- **Triggers** cause asthma attacks and include:
- **Chest infections** cause inflammation of the airway and worsen the asthma
- **Allergies** cause inflammation. Animal fur, feathers, dust and pollen are common allergens.
- **Medicines** such as aspirin and ibuprofen can trigger an attack
- **Mould** or **damp** can create fungus spores which trigger asthma attacks
- Environmental factors such as **pollution** irritate the airways. Common factors include cigarette smoke, smoke from fires, exhaust fumes and pollution from factories.
- **Temperature** is another environmental factor that can trigger an attack. Either extreme heat or extreme cold can irritate the airways.

Control and prevention

Method	How it works
Preventer inhaler	Reduces inflammation making the airways less sensitive to triggers.
Steroidal tablets	Reduces inflammation during flare-ups.
Avoiding triggers	Prevents the airways from becoming irritated to reduce the number of asthma attacks.
Lifestyle changes	Being healthy in general will improve the condition of the lungs and reduce inflammation making attacks less likely. Below are two specific important lifestyle changes.
Regular exercise	Strengthens respiratory muscles as well as the cardiovascular system so breathing becomes more efficient. It also helps keep weight down as being overweight puts a strain on the respiratory system.
Stopping smoking	Reduces the irritation caused by the chemicals in cigarette smoke.

Impact of Asthma on the individual

Physical	Intellectual
• Wheezing, shortness of breath and tight chest causes discomfort. • Persistent cough drains energy. • Less energy due to not enough oxygen getting into the blood.	• Children may miss school affecting their cognitive development. • Difficult to concentrate if you cannot breathe properly.
Emotional	**Social**
• Anxiety about asthma attacks. • Frustration about not being able to join in activities.	• May avoid social activities to avoid triggering an attack. • Time off school or work may disrupt relationships.

Bacterial pneumonia

Causes

- Bacterial pneumonia is caused by a bacterial infection of the lungs.
- The infection causes inflammation of the alveoli become inflamed.
- The inflammation widens the walls of the alveoli increasing the distance oxygen must diffuse over.
- The alveoli also fill with pus and other liquids which leaves less room for air.

Signs and symptoms

- Cough.
- Breathing difficulties.
- Chest pain.
- Fever.

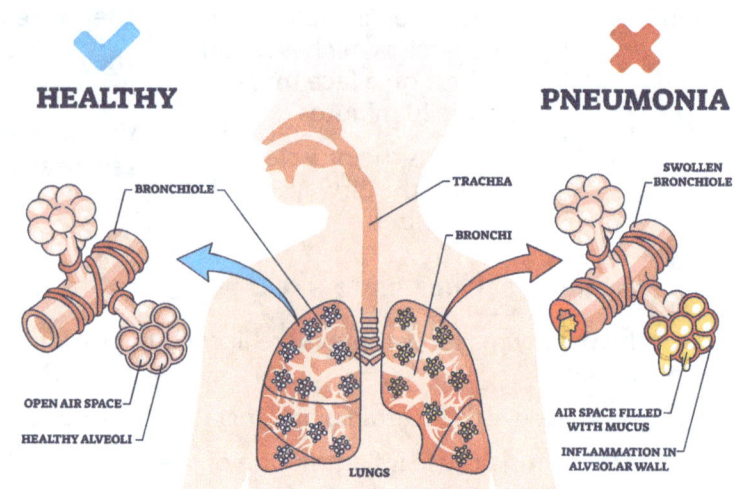

Diagnosis and monitoring

Method	Details	How and when it is used
Physical examination	A stethoscope is used to listen to the chest. Unusual sounds like crackling or wheezing can indicate an infection.	It is mostly used for diagnosis. Can be used to check infection has cleared after treatment.
X-ray	Chest x-rays can show areas of infection.	Mostly used for diagnosis. It can confirm infection and show how much of the lungs is affected.
Sputum test	Mucus (sputum) that is coughed up is sent to the lab for testing. The specific bacteria that is causing the infection can be identified and the correct antibiotics given.	It is used during diagnosis.
Blood test	Blood is tested to see how many white blood cells there are. When there are more than normal it indicates there is an infection.	Used both during diagnosis to confirm there is an infection and after treatment to confirm infection has gone.

Treatments

Treatment	How it works	Advantages	Disadvantages
Antibiotic tablets	Antibiotics contain chemicals which kill the bacterium causing the infection.	Tablets are easier to take, and the person can go home. Effective in treating the infection.	Can have side effects like nausea and vomiting. Some people have severe allergies to antibiotics.
Intravenous antibiotics	Antibiotics are given through a canula directly into a vein. Often given at the same time as fluids.	Intravenous antibiotics can be stronger and worker faster.	Patient has to remain in hospital for intravenous antibiotics.

Treatment	How it works	Advantages	Disadvantages
Fluids	Patient is encouraged to drink to prevent dehydration. Fluid can be given via a drip. Water and electrolytes are given.	Helps rehydrate a patient who feels too ill to drink.	Care must be taken not to give too much fluid.
Oxygen	Can be given through a nasal cannula, face mask or ventilator. It makes it easier for the patient to get enough oxygen.	The patient can absorb more oxygen which will make them feel better and be able to fight the infection. It will be less of a strain to breathe.	The patient will need to be treated in hospital. The mask can be uncomfortable and restricts movement and talking.

Factors making pneumonia more likely

- **Lifestyle choices** make the individual more prone to infections and make it harder for them to fight an infection. **Smoking** causes damage to the lungs which makes infections more likely.
- **Age** can affect how likely a person is to get pneumonia. Babies are more vulnerable because their immune system is not properly developed, and their airways are smaller. The elderly are more vulnerable because they have a weaker immune system and are more likely to have other conditions which increase the risk.
- **Underlying health conditions** can make people more vulnerable to the disease. **Asthma** causes damage to the lungs making them easier to infect and the steroid medication weakens the immune system. **Diabetes** also damages the immune system.
- A **weakened immune system** means that there are fewer white blood cells available to kill the infectious bacteria, so it is harder to fight the infection.

Control and prevention

Control and prevention measure	How it works
Flu vaccinations	Protects against flu which would weaken the immune system.
Lifestyle changes:	Reduce factors that make people more vulnerable to bacterial pneumonia.
Regular exercise	Strengthens immune system, improves the condition of the lungs, reduces inflammation in general which helps prevent infection.
Hydration	Helps the airways create mucus to trap bacteria so they don't infect the lungs. All body systems and cells require water to work properly, so drinking keeps the whole body in better condition.

Impact of pneumonia on the individual

Physical	Intellectual
- Always out of breath and feeling uncomfortable. - Difficulty sleeping. - Not enough energy due to lack of oxygen.	- Harder to think and concentrate. - Will not be able to go to school or work so they will miss intellectual stimulation. - Lack of oxygen can cause memory problems.
Emotional	**Social**
- Anxiety about getting another infection. - Discomfort can lead to depression or low mood.	- Too ill to socialise with anyone. - May avoid social contact if they suffer with infections regularly.

Study Tips!

- You may need to label a diagram of the respiratory system in your exam so you need to be able to recognise different structures on different pictures.
- You must be able to explain the relationship between volume and pressure in the respiratory system (the lower the volume, the higher the air pressure in the lungs) and how this is used by the body to breathe in and out.
- Understanding factors that affect rate of diffusion is important in understanding how the respiratory system works and what can go wrong with various diseases. The distance the air needs to travel (across membranes), surface area for absorption of oxygen into the blood and maintaining a diffusion gradient between the alveoli and the blood are all important factors in gas exchange.
- It is very important that you understand that the reason we breathe is to get oxygen to make energy. Some people make the mistake of saying that we need oxygen to breathe. It is the opposite way round – we breathe to get oxygen.
- You will need to be able to recommend which treatments are best for a specific person based on the advantages and disadvantages of each treatment and the circumstances of the individual.
- You need to understand the difference between a direct cause and a factor that makes a condition more likely. Factors that made a condition more likely do not guarantee that a person will develop the condition.
- When thinking about how a condition like asthma or bacteria pneumonia impact on a person, you will need to take their personal circumstances into account rather than just talk in general terms as we have done here.
- It is important to remember that bacterial pneumonia is just one type of pneumonia, and not all pneumonia is caused by bacteria. This is important when deciding on the best treatment for it.

Important terms!

Air pressure – The pressure of the air caused by the weight of the atmosphere pressing down or by the air molecules pressing against objects.

Diffuse – A natural process of molecules in a gas or a liquid where the particles move from an area of high concentration to an area of low concentration.

Mitochondria - Structure within a cell where energy is made during aerobic respiration. More active cells will have more of them. The singular for mitochondria is mitochondrion. So, you have one mitochondrion or several mitochondria.

Inflammation – Natural response to an infection within the body. The affected area swells and may look red and feel hot. This is due to more blood flowing to the area to fight infection and heal any damaged tissues.

Constrict – The word used to describe the narrowing of a biological tube by contraction of smooth muscles. This can include the narrowing of blood vessels and airways.

Dilate – Widening of any biological tube including a blood vessel or an airway.

Allergens – Any substance that triggers an immune response. Common allergens include dust mites, animal fur, peanuts, latex and some medications.

Bacterial infection – An infection of the body by bacteria.

Rehydrate – To restore the body's water content when you have lost water through sweating, bleeding or not drinking enough.

Repolarisation – When neurones get back to their normal state (resting potential) where they are ready to send an impulse. It is called repolarisation because when in this state there is a difference in charge between the outside and inside of the neurone membrane.

Nasal cannula – A flexible tube which goes across the bottom of the nose. It has two small tubes which go from the main tube into each nostril. It is used to give oxygen to a patient without using a face mask.

Ventilator – Medical device that is used to help a patient breathe. It gently pushes air into the lungs. They are often used during surgery and also if the person has a condition like pneumonia.

Recap Questions

1. What is the function of the rib cage?
2. Which muscles are involved in breathing?
3. Describe the main steps in gas exchange between the alveoli and capillaries.
4. What are mitochondria?
5. What is cellular respiration?
6. What is the role of ATP?
7. What are the main differences between aerobic and anaerobic respiration?
8. What happens during an asthma attack?
9. What is a spirometer used for?
10. How do steroidal tablets help someone with asthma?
11. What is a limitation of using a nebuliser to treat asthma?
12. Name two things that can trigger an asthma attack.
13. How can regular exercise help control asthma?
14. What happens during a bacterial pneumonia infection?
15. What physical impacts does bacterial pneumonia have on an individual?
16. What is a sputum test?
17. What is an advantage of using intravenous antibiotics to treat bacterial pneumonia?
18. Why can a flu vaccination help prevent bacterial pneumonia?

Revision Quiz

1. How can regular exercise help prevent DVT?
2. What is an atheroma?
3. In which stages of menstruation are oestrogen and progesterone levels both low?
4. Give two physical impacts of type 2 diabetes.
5. What kind of joint is the wrist?
6. Name two common symptoms of gallstones.
7. What is tachycardia?
8. Name two substances the body assimilates.
9. What is the epididymis?
10. What is homeostasis?
11. What role does the pancreas play in digestion?
12. Why might old bone cells need to be removed?
13. What is an electromyography and when might it be used?
14. What is the function of the brain stem?
15. What is a thrombectomy?

Assessment practice

1. Which is true about the cartilage in the airways of the lungs? (1)

   A The rings of cartilage in the trachea are "C" shaped

   B The rings of cartilage in the bronchi are "C" shaped

   C The rings can be narrowed to restrict air flow into the lungs

   D The rings of cartilage have cilia on them to move mucus and trapped particles away from the lungs

2. Fill in the gaps: Air will move from an area of _____ pressure to an area of _____ pressure. (2)

3. State two ways the volume of the chest cavity is increased during inspiration. (2)

4. Which is correct about the movement of carbon dioxide during gas exchange. (1)

   A Carbon dioxide moves from the alveoli into the blood

   B Carbon dioxide is moved by active transport (it is actively moved by the cells)

   C Carbon dioxide moves from the blood into the alveoli

   D Carbon dioxide in the alveoli is at a higher concentration than carbon dioxide in the blood

5. What factor is increased due to the large numbers of alveoli, which makes gas exchange as efficient as possible? (1)

6. State the name of the process of producing energy in the cells. (1)

7. Fill in the gaps: Things like dust and pollen can cause an asthma _____. These causes are known as _____. (2)

8. State two reasons why airways are narrower for people with asthma. (2)

9. What is the name of the device which measures the speed of expiration and is used to diagnose and monitor asthma? (1)

10. What is the name of the device used to listen to the lungs during breathing to help diagnose or monitor pneumonia? (1)

11. What is the correct reason why a flu vaccination helps prevent bacterial pneumonia? (1)

    A The flu virus causes the infection which leads to pneumonia

    B Fighting off flu exhausts the immune system so it cannot fight off bacterial infections of the lungs

    C The flu vaccination gets rid of the bacteria from the lungs

    D The flu vaccinate encourages the growth of "good" bacteria in the lungs

12. Being hydrated keeps the mucus thin. Explain why this helps prevent pneumonia. (2)

13. State two reasons why bacterial pneumonia can negatively affect social development. (2)

14. Describe the effect the diaphragm has on the volume of the chest cavity. (3)

15. Explain the relationship between volume and pressure during inspiration (4)

16. Explain two adaptations of the alveoli to enable gaseous exchange. (4)

17. Outline the process of anaerobic respiration in the body. (3)

18. Analyse the triggers of an asthma attack. (6)

19. Explain the use of sputum tests to diagnose bacterial pneumonia (3)

    Max is 79 years old. He lives by himself, does not exercise much and smokes.

20. Discuss methods he could use to reduce the risk of developing bacterial pneumonia. (9)

    Ben (10) lives with his parents who live in a flat in the centre of Manchester near a busy road. Both Ben's parents smoke. They have a cat named Tiger.

21. Analyse how Ben and his family can manage his condition and make asthma attacks less likely (6)

3: Digestive system

3.1 Structure and function of the digestive system

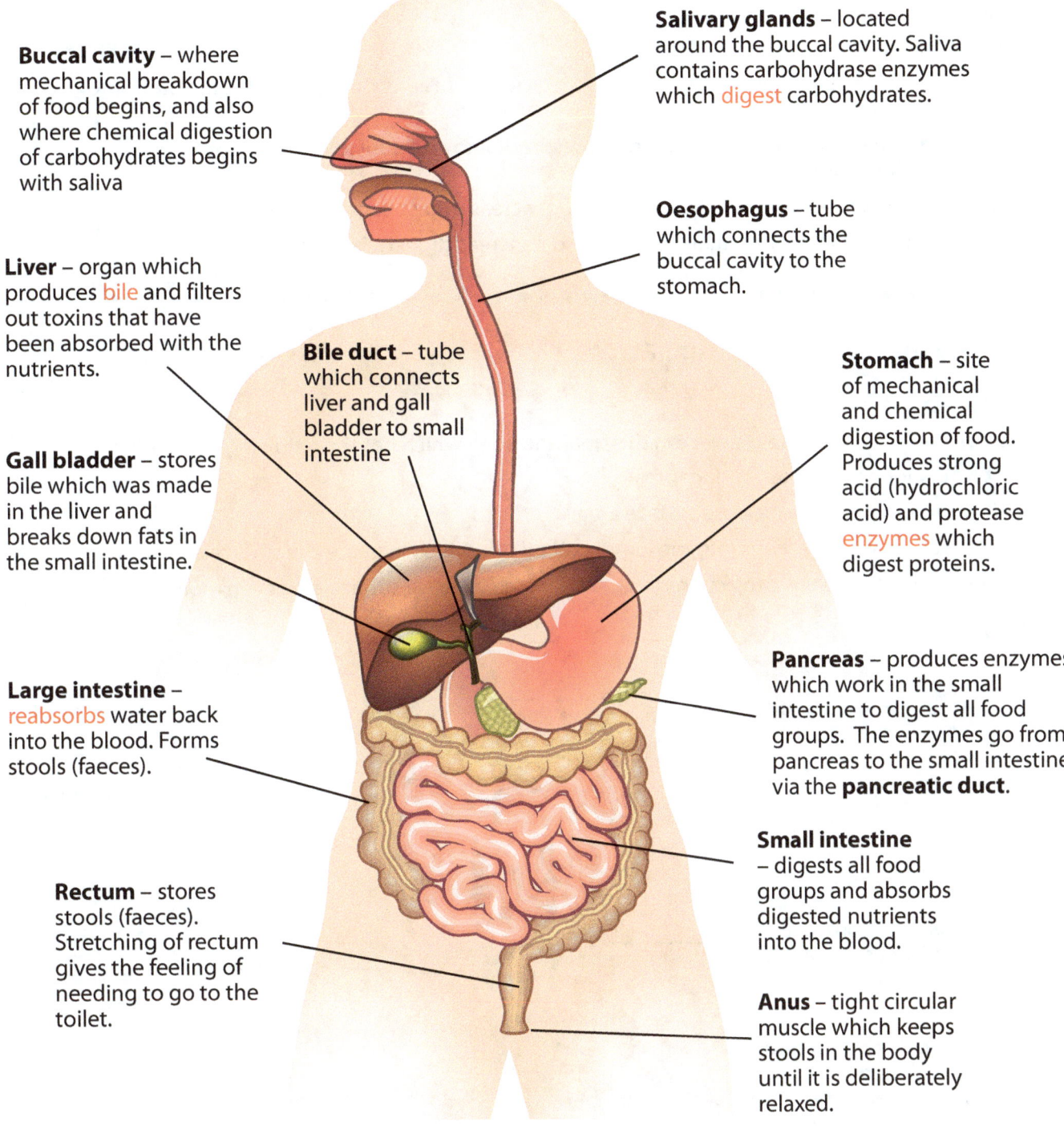

Buccal cavity – where mechanical breakdown of food begins, and also where chemical digestion of carbohydrates begins with saliva

Liver – organ which produces bile and filters out toxins that have been absorbed with the nutrients.

Gall bladder – stores bile which was made in the liver and breaks down fats in the small intestine.

Bile duct – tube which connects liver and gall bladder to small intestine

Large intestine – reabsorbs water back into the blood. Forms stools (faeces).

Rectum – stores stools (faeces). Stretching of rectum gives the feeling of needing to go to the toilet.

Salivary glands – located around the buccal cavity. Saliva contains carbohydrase enzymes which digest carbohydrates.

Oesophagus – tube which connects the buccal cavity to the stomach.

Stomach – site of mechanical and chemical digestion of food. Produces strong acid (hydrochloric acid) and protease enzymes which digest proteins.

Pancreas – produces enzymes which work in the small intestine to digest all food groups. The enzymes go from pancreas to the small intestine via the **pancreatic duct**.

Small intestine – digests all food groups and absorbs digested nutrients into the blood.

Anus – tight circular muscle which keeps stools in the body until it is deliberately relaxed.

3.2 Mechanical and chemical digestion

Mechanical digestion
- In the **mouth** – chewing breaks food into smaller pieces so that digestive enzymes can work on it more easily.
- In the **stomach** – food is churned and mixed with digestive juices.

Chemical digestion

In the mouth:
- **Carbohydrase enzymes** in the saliva break down carbohydrates into smaller carbohydrates.

In the stomach:
- **Protease enzymes** break down proteins into amino acids. Strong acid helps the enzymes work better.

In the small intestine:
- Bile from the liver/gall bladder neutralises the acid and **breaks down large fat droplets** into smaller ones.
- **Carbohydrase enzymes** from the small intestine lining and pancreas **break down carbohydrates into glucose**.
- **Protease enzymes** from small intestine and pancreas **digest proteins** into amino acids.
- **Lipase enzymes** from the small intestine and pancreas **digests fats** into fatty acids and glycerol.

3.3 Absorption and assimilation

Absorption

Absorption of nutrients takes place in the small intestine which has the following adaptations:
- It is very long to increase surface area.
- It has internal folds to increase surface area.
- The walls have projections into the lumen, called villi, which increase the surface area.
- The villi cells have tiny projections (microvilli) which increase surface area even more.

Villi

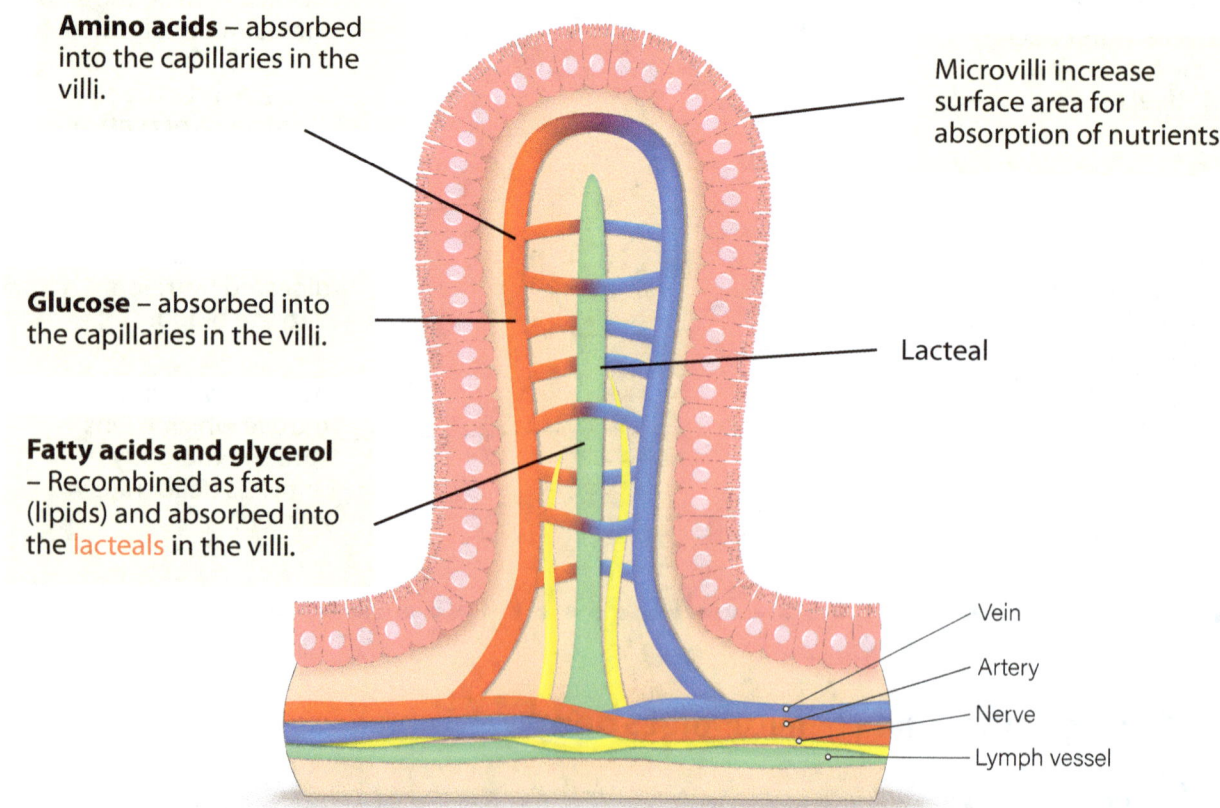

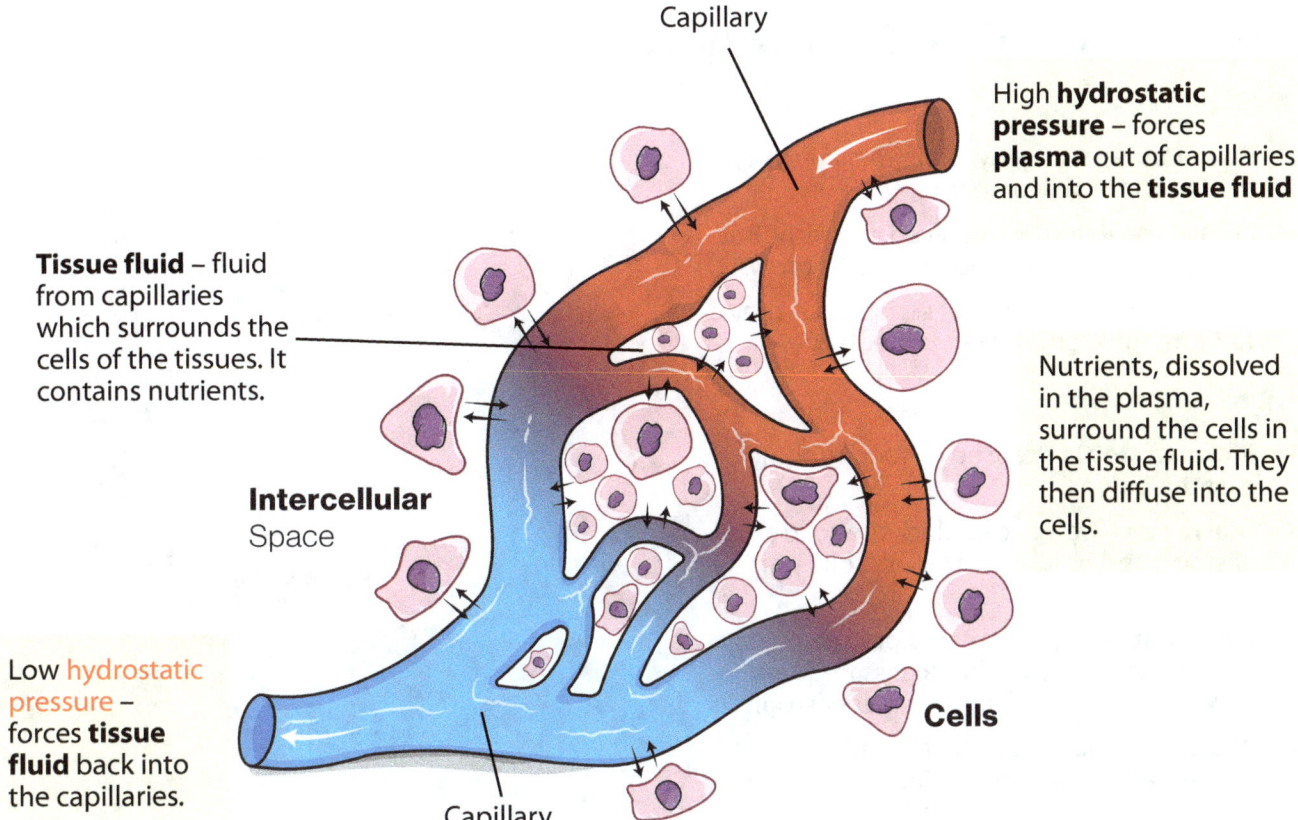

Assimilation

Assimilation is the process of changing the nutrients into substances needed by the body. Each nutrient has specific uses in the body:

Nutrient	Uses in the body
Glucose	Used for energy in cellular respiration
Amino acids	Reassembled into proteins needed by the body for: • Growth. • Repair. • Enzymes. • Hormones. • Energy in cellular respiration.
Fat	Uses include: • Component of cell walls. • Used as an energy store. • Used to make some hormones. • Energy in cellular respiration.
Vitamins	Uses vary depending on the vitamin for example: • Vitamin A – healthy immune system, healthy skin, vision. • Vitamin C – healthy immune system. Protects against cell damage. • Vitamin D – helps the body absorb calcium for the bones • Vitamin B12 – Needed to make red blood cells, important in energy production.
Minerals	Uses vary depending on the mineral for example: • Calcium – needed for teeth and bones, muscle contraction. • Iron – needed for haemoglobin in red blood cell production. • Sodium – needed for nerve and muscle function and fluid balance.

3.4 Conditions of the digestive system

Bowel polyps

- **Bowel polyps** are growths in the lining of the large intestine or rectum.
- Cells of the lining are replaced regularly. But a polyp can appear if too many cells grow.
- Polyps themselves are not serious. But they can turn into cancer if left untreated.

Signs and symptoms

- **Blood in stools** – caused by food rubbing past the polyps.
- **Diarrhoea** – polyps can block the solid part of stools and only allow the less solid parts through.
- **Constipation** – polyps can block the passage of stools, leading to less frequent bowel movements and harder, drier stools.
- **Abdominal pain** – blockages and inflammation can cause pain.

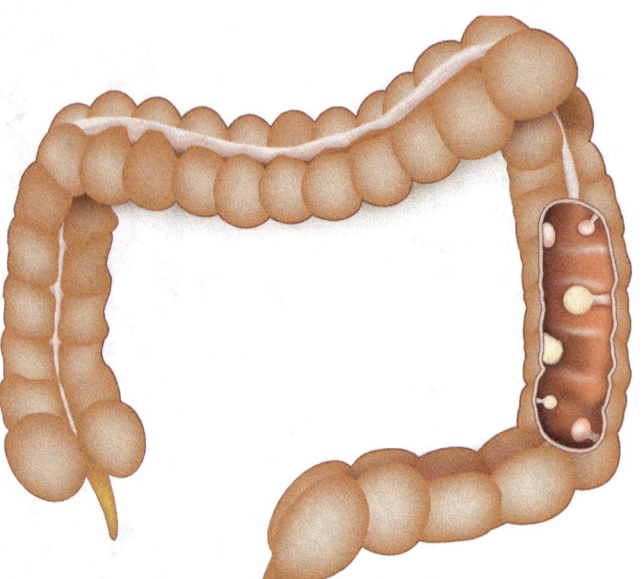

Bowel polyps

Diagnosis and monitoring

- **Screening** – Adults over 50 in the UK are sent kits to collect stool samples so they can be examined by a laboratory. Those with unusual results will be investigated further.
- **Colonoscopy** – This is a procedure where a camera is inserted into the large intestine via the anus in order to see if bowel polyps are present.

Treatments

- **Polypectomy** – This is when a wire loop is placed around the polyp and then tightened, cutting the polyp off. If required, this procedure normally takes place as the same time as a colonoscopy.
- **Open surgery** – Surgery is needed for larger polyps and involves cutting into the large intestine or rectum.

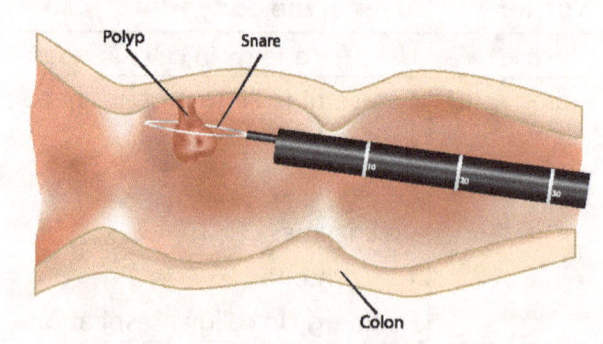

A polypectomy

Treatment	Benefits of treatment	Limitations of treatment
Polypectomy	• Simple procedure and quick recovery time. • Removes the need for surgery. • Can take place at same time as colonoscopy, so polyps are removed as soon as they are discovered.	• Only suitable for smaller or less complex polyps. • The procedure can accidentally perforate the large intestine. • Less precise than surgery.
Open surgery	• The surgeon can be very precise. • Suitable for large or complex polyps.	• Much longer recovery time. • All surgery carries additional risks.

Factors that make bowel polyps more likely

- Bowel polyps are slightly **more common in men**.
- **Being over 50** increases the risk, as there has been more time for the passage of food to damage the large intestine or rectum.
- A diet that is **high in fact and processed food**. These foods can cause inflammation which can damage the lining of the bowel.
- A diet that is **low in fibre**, as fibre can help regulate the movement of waste through the bowel.
- Genetic factors can make bowel polyps more likely, so **family history** of the condition increases the risk of developing it.
- Someone with Crohn's disease is more likely to develop bowel polyps, because it involves long-term inflammation which can damage tissue and cause polyps.
- The chemicals in cigarettes can damage the lining of the bowel, meaning **smokers** are more likely to develop bowel polyps.

Control and prevention

There are a number of **lifestyle changes** which can help prevent bowel polyps.

- **High-fibre diet**. Fibre stimulates the regular movement of the bowel, meaning there is less pressure on it and harmful substances are removed from the body more rapidly.
- **A healthy weight**.
  - » Being overweight leads to inflammation in the cells of the body, which can lead to polyps.
  - » Losing weight also reduces insulin levels, which in turn reduces the risk of polyps.
  - » Fat tissue produces hormones which can encourage the development of polyps.
- **Regular exercise**.
  - » Regular exercise reduces inflammation, which reduces the risk of bowel polyps.
  - » Exercise also encourage bowel movements which remove harmful substances from the body.
- **Stop smoking**. The harmful chemicals in cigarettes can cause bowel polyps.

Impact of the condition on the individual

Physical	Intellectual
• Polyps themselves can cause discomfort and pain. • Constipation or diarrhoea due to polyps can also be uncomfortable or painful. • Long-term blood loss from bleeding polyps can cause tiredness and fatigue.	• Any pain can distract people from their day-to-day work or activities. • People may find it hard to concentrate if they are worried about the polyps developing into cancer.
Emotional	**Social**
• People may be worried and anxious about the possibility of polyps developing into cancer. • Constipation or diarrhoea can also cause upset or frustration. • They may be embarrassed about the intimate location of the polyps.	• Appointments may impact on work or social life. • People may be reluctant to play sport or go out with friends if they are suffering constipation or diarrhoea.

Gallstones

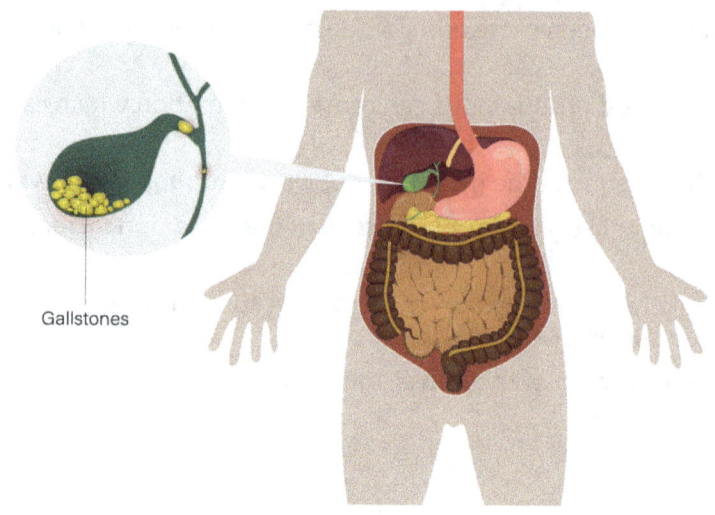

Gallstones

Causes
- Crystals of either cholesterol or bilirubin forms from the bile.
- They gradually get bigger
- They can block the bile duct.
- They prevent bile getting into the small intestine.

Signs and symptoms
- Pain in the abdomen
- Jaundice – build up of bilirubin in blood causing yellow skin and eyes.
- Fever due to infection of gall bladder or pancreas.
- Nausea

Diagnosis and monitoring

- **Physical examination** – to feel for signs of inflammation and to see if it hurts when the patient breathes in while they press at the top right of the abdomen.
- **Ultrasound scan** – to show up gallstones in the gall bladder or bile ducts.
- **Blood test** – to look for signs of infection or to do a liver function test to see how well the liver is working.

Treatments

- **Laparoscopic cholecystectomy** – removal of the gallbladder using keyhole surgery using an instrument known as a laparoscope.
- **Open cholecystectomy** – Removal of the gallbladder using open surgery.
- **Pain relief** – Pain killing medication to ease the pain.

Treatment	Benefits of treatment	Limitations of treatment
Laparoscopic cholecystectomy	• Quick recovery from surgery. • Smaller scars. • Less risk of infection.	• Possible damage to surrounding tissue. • Can cause bleeding • Not suitable for some patients such as if they have scarring from previous surgery.
Open cholecystectomy	• It is easier for the surgeon to see clearly. • Complications will be spotted more easily. • More suitable for unusual gallstones.	• Longer recovery time. • More pain due to surgery. • Higher risk of infection or excessive bleeding.
Pain relief	• Much less risk than surgery.	• It has no effect on the gallstones. • Not everyone can take painkillers, particularly people with liver problems. • They may not be enough to relieve the pain in some people.

Factors that make gallstones more likely

- Being **female** because oestrogen increases cholesterol levels.
- Being **over forty** because bile becomes more concentrated and likely to form crystals as we get older.
- Being **obese** as that increases cholesterol levels and slows the emptying of the gall bladder.
- Having a **family history** as certain genes affect the composition of bile making gallstones easier to form.
- **Alcohol abuse** because the liver is too busy detoxifying the alcohol to make bile properly.

Control and prevention

Lifestyle changes are needed to prevent gallstone formation or prevent them getting bigger and include:

- Changes to the **diet** to include high fibre, low-fat foods.
- **Losing weight** to reduce cholesterol levels and speed up emptying of the gall bladder.

Impact of the condition on the individual

Physical	Intellectual
• Severe pain. • Nausea. • Vomiting. • Weight loss.	• Distracted from intellectual activities due to pain and discomfort. • Need to miss work or education for medical appointments.
Emotional	**Social**
• Anxiety about the condition. • Depression caused by pain and discomfort. • Difficulty adjusting to lifestyle changes such as avoiding certain foods.	• More likely to avoid social contact due to pain and discomfort. • May miss social activities due to the need to attend medical appointments.

Study Tips!

- Remember that the right side of the body is on the left side of a diagram. So the liver is on the left side of the page but is actually on the right side of your body.
- The word **structure** means the physical characteristics such as what a body part looks like, what it is made of or how its tissues are arranged.
- The word **function** refers to what the body part does, what its role is.
- Use the scientific meaning of words such as **digest** rather than its everyday use. i.e. digest means to mechanically and chemically break down large molecules into smaller molecules that can be absorbed by the body.
- Remember that more food is digested in the small intestine than in the stomach.
- Words that end in "-ase" are enzymes. The part before this ending indicates what molecule the enzyme works on. So, protease enzymes break down proteins.
- It is important that you remember which enzyme digests which food molecule as enzymes are very specific on what they work on.
- Surfaces of the body which absorb substances usually have as big a surface area as possible to make absorption easier. Two examples are the respiratory system and the digestive system.
- Remember that the term "obese" is used in health and social care to refer to people with a body mass index (BMI) of 30 or above.

Important terms!

Digest – The process of breaking larger food molecules into smaller molecules so they can be absorbed into the blood.

Bile – A substance made in the liver from cholesterol bilirubin. It is used to break down fat drops into smaller drops and neutralises acid in the small intestine.

Enzyme – Biological catalyst which speeds up reactions in the body.

Digestive juice – Fluid found in the digestive system which contains enzymes that are used to break down food molecules.

Reabsorb – Process by which substances (in this case water) are taken back into the body.

Amino acid – An organic molecule which is a building block of proteins. There are 20 different amino acids. The order in which they combine with each other determines the type of protein that is made.

Fatty acid – A part of a fat molecule, fatty acid is a long chain of carbon and hydrogen atoms with a carboxyl group (COOH) at one end. Fat molecules are made of one molecule of glycerol and three molecules of fatty acid.

Glycerol – A type of alcohol with three carbon atoms. It forms the backbone of fat molecules when three fatty acid molecules attach to it.

Lumen – The name given to the inside space inside any biological tube such as the digestive system or a blood vessel.

Villi/villus – A villus is a small projection from the walls of the small intestine into the lumen of the digestive system. It helps increase the surface area for absorption of nutrients. The plural of villus is villi.

Microvilli – Tiny projections from the cells of villi which extend into the lumen of the small intestine. They increase the surface area of the villi.

Lacteal – Vessel like a capillary which is part of the lymphatic system.

Hydrostatic pressure – Force of blood on the walls of blood vessels caused by the pumping of the heart.

Cholesterol – A type of fat found in the body. It helps form bile. It can build up in bile and cause gallstones.

Bilirubin – A yellow substance produced when red blood cells are broken down. It helps form bile.

Oestrogen – Hormone of the female reproductive system.

Detoxify – The process by which the liver breaks down alcohol in the blood to reduce its toxic effects on the body.

Laparoscope – A medical instrument consisting of a long flexible tube with a light and camera at one end. It is inserted into the abdominal cavity through a small cut to help diagnose various conditions and carry out keyhole surgery.

Recap Questions

1. What is the role of the gall bladder?
2. What happens during the chemical digestion of proteins?
3. Where does mechanical digestion take place?
4. What is assimilation?
5. What role does hydrostatic pressure have in assimilation?
6. What is a gallstone made of?
7. What is jaundice?
8. Give two lifestyle changes that can help reduce the risk of bowel polyps.
9. Name a surgical treatment for gallstones.
10. Why is a heavy drinker of alcohol at greater risk of gallstones?
11. Why is being female a risk factor for gallstones?
12. Give an emotional impact on an individual of having gallstones.
13. What is a colonoscopy?

Revision Quiz

1. Describe two emotional impacts of developing angina.
2. What do capillaries do?
3. Give one emotional impact of osteoarthritis on an individual.
4. Why are older people more likely to develop DVT?
5. Where in the body are the quadriceps?
6. What is endometrial tissue?
7. What is a negative feedback mechanism?
8. What happens to the diaphragm during expiration?
9. What role does inflammation play in asthma?
10. What are the disadvantages of treating bacterial pneumonia with oxygen?
11. Give one physical impact of carpal tunnel syndrome.
12. What is type 2 diabetes?
13. What is the function of the pituitary gland?

Assessment practice

1. Identify the components A-C in the diagram below. (3)

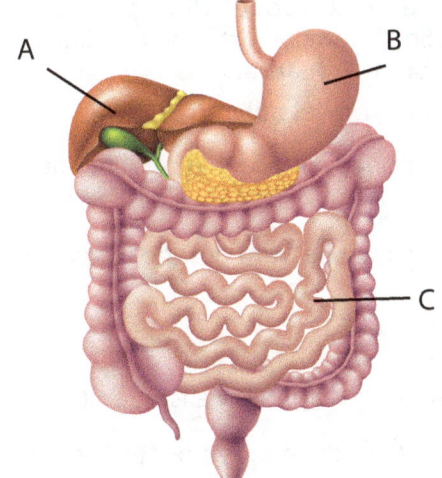

Letter	Part of digestive system
A	
B	
C	

2. Enzymes are produced by the walls of the small intestine. Which other part of the digestive system produces enzymes which act in the small intestine? (1)

3. Protease is an enzyme which digests proteins. State two other enzymes found in the digestive system. (2)

4. Chewing is an example of mechanical digestion. State one other part of the digestive system where mechanical digestion takes place. (1)

5. Which part of the digestive system is responsible for absorption of nutrients into the blood? (1)

   A Stomach   **C** Large intestine
   B Liver   **D** Small intestine

6. Lars has eaten a bacon sandwich. Explain what happens to the protein in the sandwich before it is absorbed into the blood. (3)

7. Explain how the small intestine is adapted to absorb nutrients. (3)

8. Describe bile and its role in the digestive system. (3)

9. One use of fat in the body is to provide energy. State one other use of fats in the body. (1)

10. Identify which substances are absorbed into structures A and B in the diagram of the small intestine. (2)

11. Analyse how bowel polyps affect the digestive system. (6)

12. Outline how colonoscopy is used to detect bowel polyps. (3)

13. Fill in the gaps about the treatment of bowel polyps by polypectomy. (4)

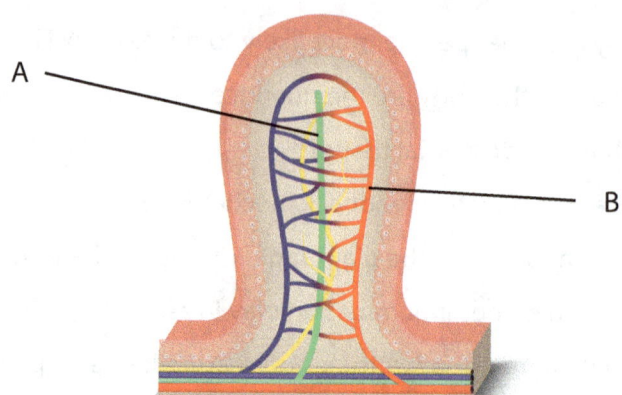

A _____ is inserted into the bowel through the anus. When a polyp is located a _____ _____ is placed over the polyp and tightened. This cuts off the polyp which can then be sent to the laboratory to check for _____.

14. State two limitations of open surgery to remove polyps. (2)

15. Outline measures that can be used to prevent bowel polyps. (3)

Suzanne is 52 years old. She owns her own hair dressing business which gives her little time to cook so she often eats ready meals and takeaways. She smokes about 15-20 cigarettes a day. She has just been diagnosed with bowel polyps. She is familiar with the condition because her aunt was diagnosed with the same thing about 10 years ago.

16. Discuss reasons why Suzanne is at higher risk of developing bowel polyps. (9)

17. One component of bile is cholesterol. State another component of bile that might contribute to the formation of gallstones. (1)

18. Which structure can be blocked by gallstones which prevents bile from getting into the small intestine? (1)

19. Outline why gallstones can cause jaundice. (3)

20. Fill in the blanks in the following sentences about methods to diagnose gallstones. (3)

High frequency sound is used during _____ scans which creates a picture of the gallstones. Blood tests, on the other hand, look for white blood cells which indicate the presence of _____ blood cells. Certain substances can also be detected in the blood which show problems with _____ function.

21. State two advantages of laparoscopic cholecystectomy over open surgery. (2)

22. State two limitations of pain relief used as a treatment for gallstones. (2)

23. Outline why obesity increases the risk of gallstones. (3)

24. Analyse how lifestyle changes can help control gallstones. (6)

Martin is 44 years old and is a self-employed plumber. He works long hours and so tends to go out to the pub in the evening to relax and eat his meals. At work he tends to have high calory snacks to keep his energy levels high. He is about 2 stone overweight.

25. Discuss the possible impacts of gallstones on Martin's life. (9)

4: Musculoskeletal system

4.1 Skeletal system

Skeletal structure

The **axial skeleton** is the central part of the skeleton and makes up the supporting framework.

Sternum (breastbone)
Protects the heart and lungs. Connects to the ribs with cartilage.

Cranium
Part of the skull which encloses and protects the brain.

Ribs
Extend from the vertebral column and around the front of the body. Protects heart and lungs and are needed for breathing.

Vertebral column
Made of 33 bones and runs from base of skull to pelvis. Protects the spinal cord, helps with posture and movement.

The **appendicular skeleton** consists of the limbs and the bones they attach to. The main function is movement.

Clavicle (collar bone)
Connects sternum and scapula bones. Stabilises movement at the shoulder.

Humerus
Upper arm bone

Scapula (shoulder blade)
Connects humerus to clavicle. It is where should, upper back and arm muscles attach.

Radius
The lower arm bone that is on the same side as the thumb.

Ulna
The lower arm bone that is on the same side as the little finger.

Pelvis (hip bone)
Supports the upper body, protects the pelvic organs and provides attachment to leg bones and muscles.

Femur
Upper leg bone

Patella (kneecap)
Protects the knee joint and helps movement of the leg.

Fibula
Thinner of the two lower leg bones which is located towards the outside. Provides stability and supports the muscles of the lower leg.

Tibia (shin bone)
Larger of the two lower leg bones. Bears the weight of the body during standing or walking.

89

Structure of bone

Component of bone	Location	Structure	Function
Growth plates	Both ends of long bones.	Made of hyaline cartilage.	Area where new bone tissue is added to allow for children and adolescents to grow.
Compact bone	Outer layer of bones.	Tightly packed bone tissue containing bone cells, collagen fibres and minerals.	Provides strength.
Bone marrow	In the hollow section of long bones and in spaces of spongy bones.	Consists of red and yellow bone marrow.	Red bone marrow makes all blood cells. Yellow bone marrow stores fat but can become red bone marrow when needed.
Cartilage	At the ends of bones in the joints, tip of the nose, the outer ear and as part of the rib cage.	More flexible, softer and smoother than bone.	Used to give the rib cage elasticity during breathing. Helps bones move against each other smoothly at the joint.

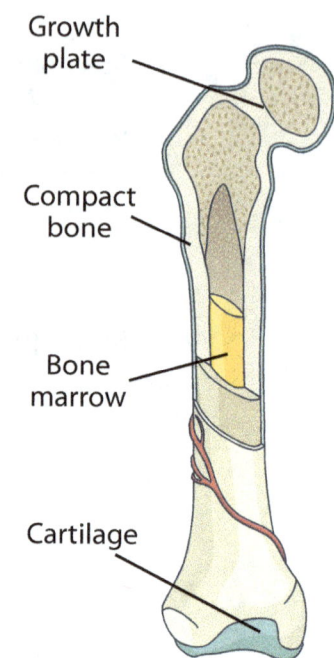

Formation of bone

Bone changes in thickness and can mend when broken. It can do this because it has two types of cell within the bone:

- **Osteoclasts** break down bone. It does this to break down broken bits of bone before mending or to release some calcium if needed by the body.
- **Osteoblasts** lay down new bone. It will do this if bones need to be stronger, during growth, and when mending broken bone.

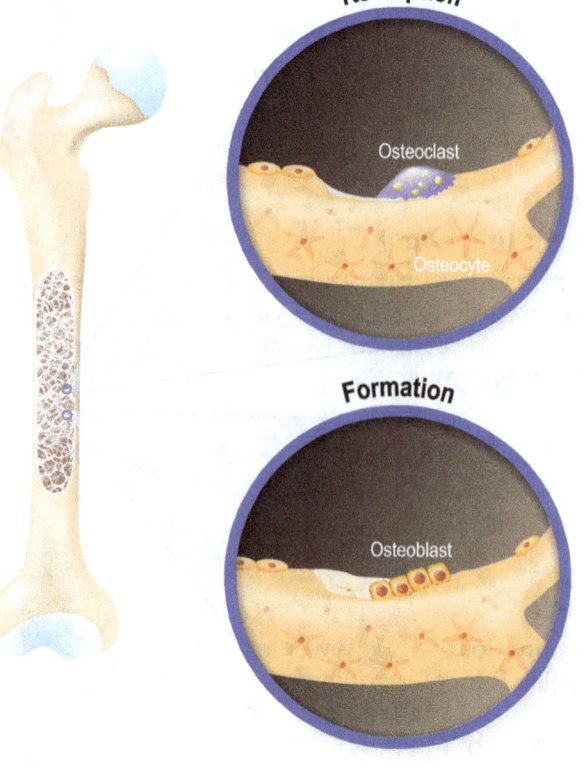

Synovial joints

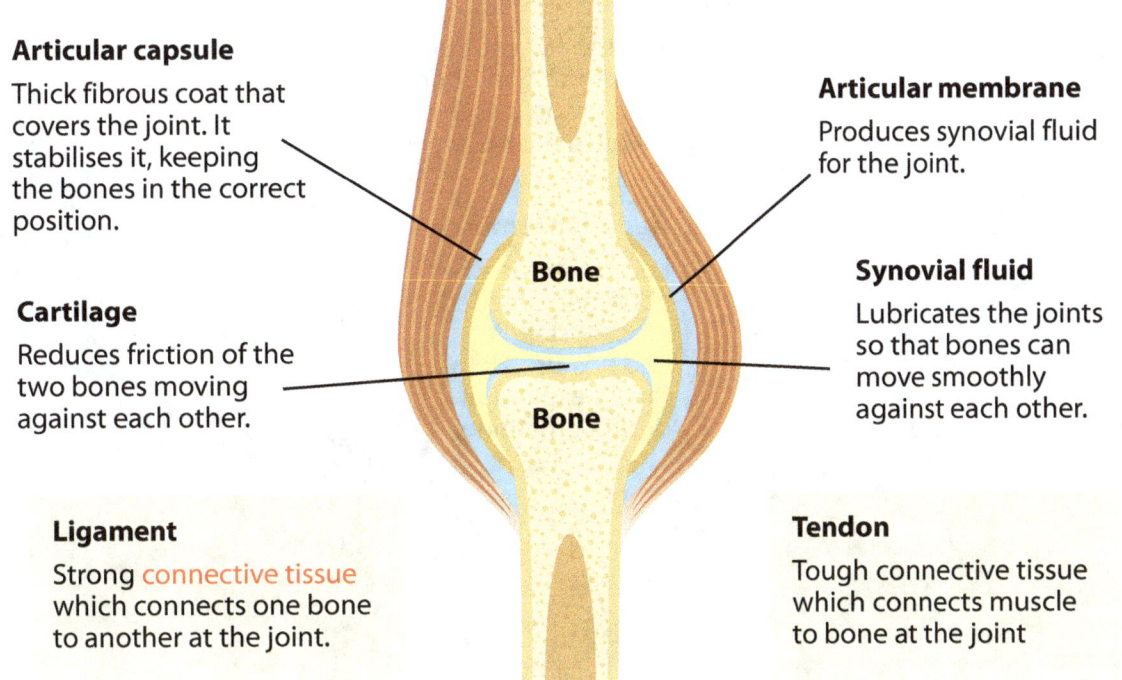

Articular capsule
Thick fibrous coat that covers the joint. It stabilises it, keeping the bones in the correct position.

Cartilage
Reduces friction of the two bones moving against each other.

Articular membrane
Produces synovial fluid for the joint.

Synovial fluid
Lubricates the joints so that bones can move smoothly against each other.

Ligament
Strong connective tissue which connects one bone to another at the joint.

Tendon
Tough connective tissue which connects muscle to bone at the joint

Types of joints

Type of joint	Description	Examples in the body
Pivot	Allows rotation around an axis.	• In the neck between the first and second vertebrae. • In the wrist to allow the radius and ulna to cross over each other.
Hinge	Allows movement on one plane like in a door hinge.	• Elbow. • Knee.
Ball and socket	Allows a bone to move in most directions.	• Shoulder – arm can move in any direction. • Hip – a bit less movement but more stability.
Saddle	A convex bone fits into an indentation in another bone like someone sitting on a saddle.	• At the base of the thumb.
Gliding/sliding	Allows bones to slide against each other along a flat or almost flat surface.	• The bones of the wrist. • The bones of the ankle.
Condyloid	An oval-shaped bone fitting into an oval-shaped cavity in another bone. Allows good movement but no rotation.	• Wrist – allows side-to-side movement. • Ankle – allowing mostly up and down movements with a small amount of side to side.

4: Musculoskeletal system

4.2 Muscular system

Deltoids
Run over the shoulder joints. Pulls arms away from the body at the shoulders, so that you can hold arms out to the side.

Pectorals
Run across the chest. Pulls arms across the body. Brings shoulders towards each other. Helps in pushing movements.

Abdominal muscles
Located across the abdomen. Needed for core stability and posture. Helps forced expiration during breathing.

Triceps
Run up the back of the upper arm. Pulls lower arm back down away from the shoulder. Straightens the arm.

Biceps
Connects shoulder to just below the elbow. Pulls lower arm up towards the shoulder.

Quadriceps
Found at the front of the thigh. Straightens the legs during walking and running. Helps flex the hips.

Gastrocnemius
Also called the calf muscle. Helps bend the knee and point the toes.

Hamstrings
Found at the back of the thigh. Bends the legs during walking and running. Helps stabilise the knee joint during standing.

4.3 Conditions of the musculoskeletal system

Carpal tunnel syndrome

Causes

The **carpal tunnel** is a gap between the bones in the wrists through which the **median nerve** runs. The gap can become narrower and compresses the nerve. This stops messages get through the nerve to and from the hand leading to the symptoms.

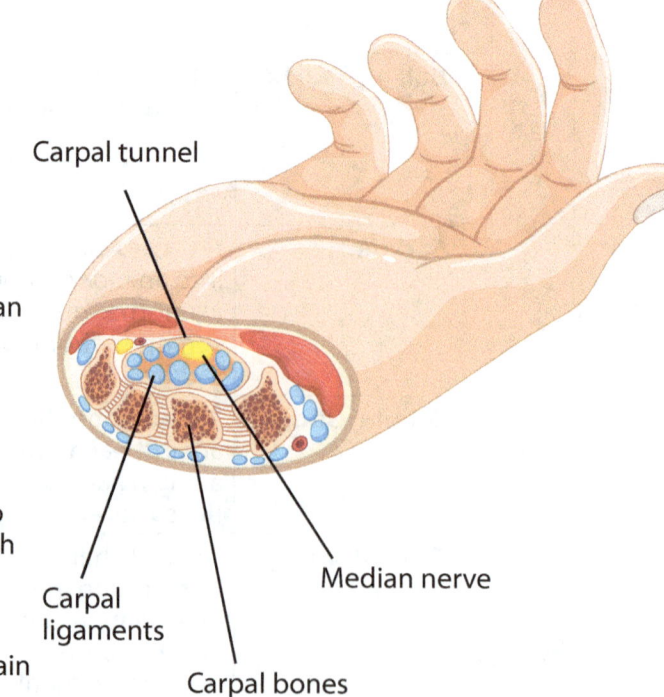

Signs and symptoms

- Numbness in the hands as messages are struggling to travel along the median nerve from the hands through the carpal tunnel to the brain.
- Tingling in the hands.
- Pain in the arms and hands due to the swelling and pain messages from the median nerve.
- Weakness in the hands and wrists as messages cannot get through the median nerve to the muscles in the hand.

Diagnosis and monitoring

Method	Details	How and when it is used
Physical examination	The doctor will check if the wrist is swollen. They will press on the carpal tunnel to see if symptoms get worse. If the patient holds their hands in a flexed position, it will often cause tingling in the hands.	This is usually the first test carried out. It will help the doctor decide if further tests are needed.
Ultrasound	High frequency sound is used to make a picture of the wrist. Can be used to detect and measure swelling around the median nerve.	Can be used if other tests are unclear. Used to guide surgery and used to check whether treatments are working.
Electromyography nerve test	The electrical activity of the median nerve is tested with electrodes. It can detect if the nerve is working properly.	Can also be used when other tests are unclear.

Treatments

Surgical treatment	Non-surgical treatments
Carpal tunnel surgery	Wrist splints
	Pain medication
	Hand exercises

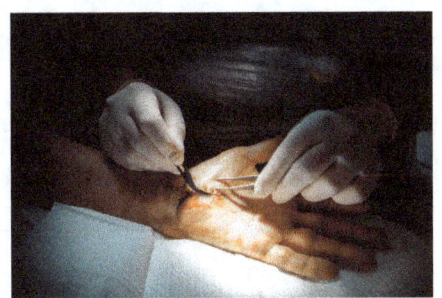

- In carpal tunnel surgery (upper photo), the carpal ligament which forms part of the carpal tunnel, is cut to reduce the pressure on the median nerve.
- Wrist splints (lower photo) keep the wrist in a position where there is less pressure on the median nerve.
- Pain medication can include NSAID medication like ibuprofen or corticosteroids. They can be used to relieve pain short term.
- Hand exercises relieve pressure on the wrist. They include stretching and muscle strengthening exercises.

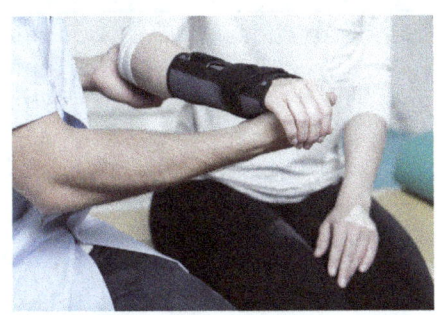

Treatment	Advantages	Disadvantages
Carpal tunnel surgery	• Permanent solution. • Improve symptoms straight away. • Quick recovery – patient can often go home the same day.	• Risk of infection due to cuts. • It may take a month to get full use of hand back after surgery.
Wrist splints	• Non-invasive option which does not have the same risks as surgery. • Does not require drugs.	• Can lead to weakness in the muscles as they are not being used as much. • Only useful for quite mild symptoms.
Pain medication	• Can ease the pain and allow the person to carry on their life.	• Often the pain killers are not strong enough. • It does not treat the problem
Hand exercises	• They can help ease the pressure and the discomfort. • Can be used to delay the need for surgery. • Can be used alongside pain killers and use of a splint.	• They will not work if they are not done properly. • They are not effective in severe cases.

Factors making carpal tunnel syndrome more likely

- **Wrist fractures** can cause swelling and scar tissue which narrows the carpal tunnel.
- **Obesity** and being **overweight** leads to fluid retention and inflammation which narrow the carpal tunnel.
- **Family history** of the condition can mean you are genetically more likely to develop carpal tunnel syndrome.
- **Working with vibrating tools** causes the wrist to vibrate which can cause damage and inflammation of the wrist which narrows the carpal tunnel.
- **Rheumatoid arthritis** is a condition affecting joints where the body's own immune system attacks the joint. The inflammation caused by the rheumatoid arthritis narrows the carpal tunnel.
- **Hormone changes** can cause swelling. Changes in hormones during pregnancy and menopause increase fluid retention which causes the carpal tunnel to narrow. Excess thyroid hormones also cause swelling in the area.

Control and prevention

Method	How it works
Grip with less force	Gripping strongly strains the muscles and tendons that make up part of the carpal tunnel. So, gripping with less force will make inflammation less likely.
Take breaks when working with hands	Taking breaks is particularly important if you do repetitive movements with your hands such as computer work. The break gives the wrist time to recover before it is put under strain again.
Keep hands warm	Cold temperatures increases stiffness in the wrist and slows blood flow. These make carpal tunnel symptoms worse. Keeping hands warm should reduce this.
Hand stretches	Hand stretches reduce tension in the wrist and opens the carpal tunnel. This reduces pressure on the median nerve and eases symptoms.

Impact of carpal tunnel syndrome on the individual

Physical	Intellectual
• Pain causes discomfort. • Discomfort gets worse at night and affects sleep. • Can weaken grip making it hard to carry out day-to-day activities.	• Pain can make it hard to focus. • May need to take time off work and miss out on intellectual stimulation.

Emotional	Social
• Frustration due to difficulty in carrying out day-to-day tasks. • Anxiety about operation.	• May not be able to join in social activities. • May withdraw due to difficulties. • May become dependent on others causing feelings of guilt and possible conflict.

Osteoarthritis

Osteoarthritis is a condition which affects the joints.

Causes

- Cartilage that covers the ends of the bones at the joint wears away.
- The space between the end of one bone and the end of the other reduces.
- This causes friction between the bones when they move against each other.
- The friction causes inflammation which causes tissue to swell and become painful.
- The damage to bones causes them to grow unevenly and produce outgrowths called **bone spurs**.

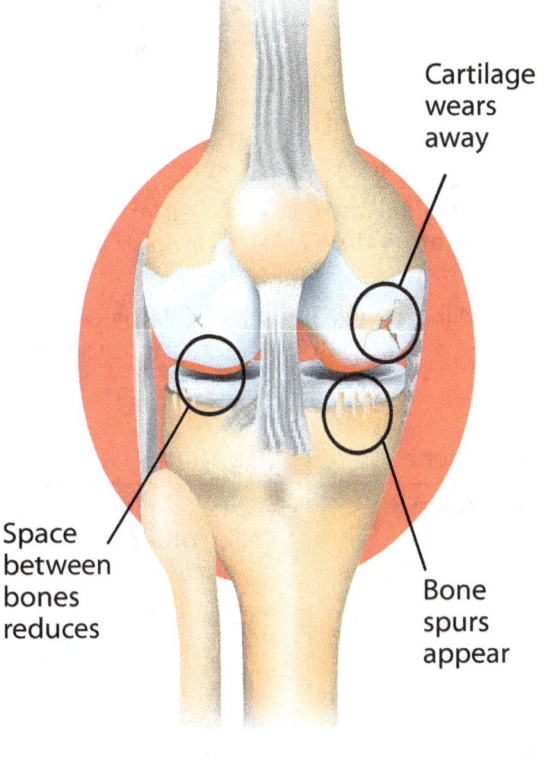

Signs and symptoms

- Pain.
- Inflammation.
- Stiffness.
- Reduced movement at the affected joints.
- Grating sounds at the joints as bones rub together.

Diagnosis and monitoring

Method	Details	How and when it is used
Physical examination	The doctor will look for inflammation (redness and swelling). They will watch while the patient moves the joint to see the range of movement. They will feel for bone spurs.	A physical examination is the first stage of the diagnosis. The doctor may send the patient for further tests.
X-ray	X-rays can show worn cartilage and bone spurs. The ends of the bones in affected joints will be denser- this shows as whiter areas on the X-ray.	Used for people over 45 whose joint pain gets worse if they move the joint more. It is used to confirm the diagnosis and to monitor if the condition is getting worse.
Exploratory surgery	A small cut is made over the joint and an arthroscope is inserted. The camera can be used to see damage to the joint.	This technique is not used often – only when other methods have been inconclusive.

Treatments

Surgical treatments	Non-surgical treatments
Joint fusing	Pain medication
Joint replacement	NSAID medication
	Steroid injections

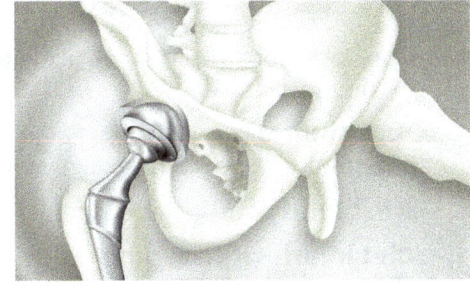

4: Musculoskeletal system

Treatment	How it works
Joint fusing	• Fuses bones at the affected joints to reduce movement and ease symptoms. More likely to be used in fingers, thumb, wrist, feet and spine.
Joint replacement	• The damaged joint is replaced with an artificial joint - see hip above.
Pain medication	• Pain medication, like paracetamol, is given to ease symptoms.
Non-steroidal anti-inflammatory drugs (NSAID)	• NSAID medication is given to reduce inflammation and ease symptoms. They also act as pain killers.
Steroid injections	• The damaged area of the joint is injected with steroids. This reduced inflammation to ease symptoms as pressure on the joints is reduced.

Treatment	Advantages	Disadvantages
Joint fusing	• Bones no longer rub against each other, so pain is reduced. • Stabilises joints.	• Loss of movement at the joint • Can restrict day-to-day activities • Surgery may require a long recovery period. • Surgery can lead to nerve damage and infections.
Joint replacement	• Movement is regained at the joint. • Pain is reduced • Replacement joints can last 15-20 years.	• Sometimes new joints fail • Long periods of physiotherapy may be needed. • The new joints do not last forever and will begin to not work properly
Pain medication	• Can ease the pain so the individual can carry on with day-to-day life. • No prescription is required for paracetamol.	• Often the pain killers are not strong enough to ease the pain. • Long-term use of pain killers can damage organs such as the liver.
Non-steroidal anti-inflammatory drugs (NSAID)	• Can be used to reduce inflammation and as a pain killer. • Some types can be obtained without a prescription.	• Must not be taken on an empty stomach as they have been associated with stomach ulcers. • Can cause kidney problems if used long term. • Can increase the risk of heart attack and stroke.
Steroid injections	• They start to ease pain within a few hours. • One injection can last for a few months.	• Steroids can cause damage to joints such as weakening tendons and ligaments. • Can only be given a few times a year due to potential damage to joints. • Sometimes the damage caused by the steroids makes the arthritis worse.

Factors making osteoarthritis more likely

- **Age** – osteoarthritis is more likely the older the person gets as they have had more wear and tear on their joints.
- **Obesity** increases the risk as being overweight puts more strain on hip and knee joints. Inflammation is also more likely when you are overweight.
- **Other joint conditions** such as rheumatoid arthritis, gout and joint laxity increase the risk.
- **Joint injuries** increase the risk of arthritis as they speed up wear and tear and cause inflammation.

Control and prevention

Method	How it works
Joint support devices	Improve the stability of the joint. Can include braces (wrist and knee) which wrap around the affected joint. They allow movement but keep the joint in line.
	Heel or shoe inserts (orthotics) ensures weight is evenly distributed if one leg is shorter due to arthritis.
Lifestyle changes	Can be used to ease symptoms or to help prevent the condition from developing.
Exercise regularly	Strengthens and stabilises the joints by strengthening the muscles around the joint. Exercise also acts as a natural pain killer.
	Exercise increases flexibility to maintain good movement at the joints.
Lose weight	Reduces the strain on the joints caused by excess weight.
	Reduces inflammation which makes the condition worse.
	Improves overall health and mental health.

Impact of osteoarthritis on the individual

Physical	Intellectual
• Can have mild to severe pain. • Can reduce mobility leading to other health problems. • Pain and inflammation will reduce energy affecting daily activities.	• Difficulty concentrating due to pain. • Poor mobility may cause the person to avoid going to places where they may get intellectual stimulation.
Emotional	**Social**
• Pain and stress can cause low mood. • Frustration caused by difficulty doing day-to-day activities. • They may feel they are a burden.	• Pain and poor mobility may mean they avoid going out to socialise. • It is easier to become socially isolated if poor mobility prevents you from going out.

Study Tips!
- You may need to label diagrams of the skeletal or muscular system with bones or muscles that are mentioned in the specification – you will not be asked to label other bones or muscles.
- Remember that minerals such as calcium are not just needed in the bones. Calcium is needed for muscles to contract and nerve impulses to cross synapses. This is why bone cells such as **osteoclasts** which break down bone are needed, so that there is enough calcium in the muscles and nerves.
- When learning about methods of diagnosing and monitoring each condition, it is important that you understand at what point in the diagnosis each method is used and how they are used when monitoring whether the condition is improving or getting worse.
- You may need to look at X-rays to determine whether an individual has osteoarthritis or not.

Important terms!

Collagen fibre – A protein fibre found in many tissues including cartilage, bone and hair to add strength.

Connective tissue – A group of tissues that are found throughout the body, are used to support or bind other tissues and usually made of both cells and non-cellular material.

Convex – A shape that bows outwards. The surface of a ball is convex.

Non-invasive – A procedure that does not involve entering the body such as through a needle or a cut for an operation.

Range of movement – How much part of the body can move in different directions. The more different directions and the more distance in those directions the body part can move, the greater the range of movement.

Orthotics – Custom designed devices that can be put inside shoes to support feet and ankle and correct problems such as having one leg longer than the other.

Arthroscope – A medical instrument used to investigate joint problems. It consists of a flexible tube with a camera and light on one end. It is inserted into a cut next to the joint so the joint structure can be seen.

Steroids – A biological molecule which is made from fat and are important in metabolism. Some act as hormones. Cholesterol is an example of a steroid.

Physiotherapy – A healthcare intervention which uses targeted exercises to regain lost abilities, improve mobility and reduce pain caused by injury or disease.

Rheumatoid arthritis – A condition which affects joints. It is an autoimmune disease caused by the person's own white blood cells attacking the joint and causing inflammation and damage.

Recap Questions

1. What is the function of the rib cage?
2. Where in a bone is cartilage found?
3. Describe the difference between osteoclasts and osteoblasts.
4. What is a ligament?
5. What is the role of the articular membrane in a synovial joint?
6. What kind of joint is at base of the thumb?
7. Where in the body would you find a hinge joint?
8. Where in the body would you find the gastrocnemius muscle?
9. What is the function of the hamstrings?
10. Why can carpal tunnel syndrome cause tingling in the hands?
11. Name one other symptom of carpal tunnel syndrome.
12. How is ultrasound used to diagnose carpal tunnel syndrome?
13. What are the advantages of using wrist splints to treat carpal tunnel syndrome?
14. Why might a pregnant woman be more prone to carpal tunnel syndrome?
15. Describe what causes osteoarthritis.
16. Give one advantage of joint fusing as a treatment for osteoarthritis.
17. Give one disadvantage of non-steroidal anti-inflammatory drugs as a treatment for osteoarthritis.
18. How can exercise help prevent osteoarthritis?
19. Describe the social impacts of osteoarthritis on an individual.
20. What is a bone spur?

Revision Quiz

1. What is a thrombolytic?
2. What hormone do the testes produce?
3. Who might be given anticoagulant medicine?
4. What is the difference between the large intestine and small intestine?
5. What two lifestyle changes can someone at risk of type 2 diabetes make?
6. What structure in the heart triggers a heartbeat?
7. Give two symptoms of menopause.
8. What is the function of the synaptic knob in a neurone?
9. What is the role of haemoglobin in breathing?
10. Give an emotional impact of testicular cancer on an individual.
11. What products are required for aerobic respiration? What substances and waste products are created?
12. What is bile?
13. What happens during the luteal phase of the menstrual cycle?
14. What are the differences between the two types of inhalers available for asthma?
15. What is the role of the central nervous system?
16. What is an MRI scan?
17. Give a physical impact of endometriosis on an individual.

Assessment practice

1. What is the name of the bone at the front of the body which the ribs attach to? (1)
2. What is the scientific name for the kneecap bone? (1)
3. Where in a bone is compact bone found? (1)
4. State two functions of cartilage. (2)
5. Fill in the gaps: _____ connect bones to each other while _____ connect muscles to bones. (2)
6. Which is **incorrect** about synovial joints? (1)

   A The synovial fluid reduces friction.
   B Ligaments help keep bones in position and prevents movements in the wrong direction.
   C There can be more than two bones in the joint.
   D The growth plate is where the articular cartilage connects to the bone.

7. State three muscles which are found in the leg. (3)
8. Fill in the gaps: The _____ are found across the chest. The _____ muscles are found in the shoulder and are used to lift the arms away from the body. (2)
9. State the name of the nerve which is affected by carpal tunnel syndrome. (1)
10. State two limitations of the use of wrist splints to treat carpal tunnel syndrome. (2)
11. Which is correct about factors which make carpal tunnel syndrome more likely? (1)

    A Wrist fractures cut the median nerve and cause the condition.
    B Being overweight increases fat tissue which presses on the median nerve.
    C Vibrating tools make the nerves in the hand less sensitive.
    D Rheumatoid arthritis is an autoimmune disease, and it causes white blood cells to attack the median nerve.

12. State two things a doctor will look for when carrying out a physical examination to diagnose osteoarthritis. (2)
13. State two limitations of joint replacement surgery. (2)
14. State two benefits of steroid injections to treat osteoarthritis. (2)
15. State two reasons why losing weight can help prevent and control osteoarthritis. (2)
16. Explain how bone is formed and repaired if broken. (4)
17. Explain the movement of the bones in a hinge joint (4)
18. Outline how muscles control the movement of the lower arm at the elbow. (4)
19. Analyse methods used to control or prevent carpal tunnel syndrome. (6)
20. Explain the use of joint fusing surgery to treat osteoarthritis. (3)
21. Amina is 88 years old and lives alone in a sheltered housing complex. She enjoys gardening and socialising with friends. Discuss possible impacts of developing osteoarthritis in her hips and hands on Amina. (9)
22. Explain the causes of the symptoms of osteoarthritis. (6)

    Jane (48) has just been diagnosed with carpal tunnel syndrome. She knows about this because her sister and mother have also been diagnosed with the condition. She works as a typist at an office near her home. She has recently been on a diet because she is two stone overweight for her height.

23. Discuss potential reasons some people are more likely to develop carpal tunnel syndrome. Suggest which reasons are most likely to relate to Jane. (9)

5: Control and regulatory systems

5.1 The nervous system

Components of the nervous system

The **central nervous system** is made up of the brain and spinal cord. Its functions are to:
- Receive and interpret information from the senses from sensory neurones.
- Sends instructions to parts of the body along **motor neurones**.
- Is responsible for thoughts, decisions, ability to communicate and memory.

The **peripheral nerves** are the nerves that extend throughout the rest of the body. It includes both sensory and motor neurones. It consists of all nerves that are not in the central nervous system.

The **autonomic nervous system** is part of the peripheral nervous system and controls functions that you are not aware of (involuntary) such as breathing rate. It consists of:
- Sympathetic nervous system which prepares the body for action.
- Parasympathetic nervous system which calms the body back down again and stimulates digestion.

The **spinal cord** is part of the central nervous system. It connects the brain to the peripheral nerves and coordinates reflex actions.

Sensory neurones carry nerve impulses (signals) from sense cells and organs to the brain or spinal cord.

Motor neurones carry nerve impulses from the brain to muscles or glands.

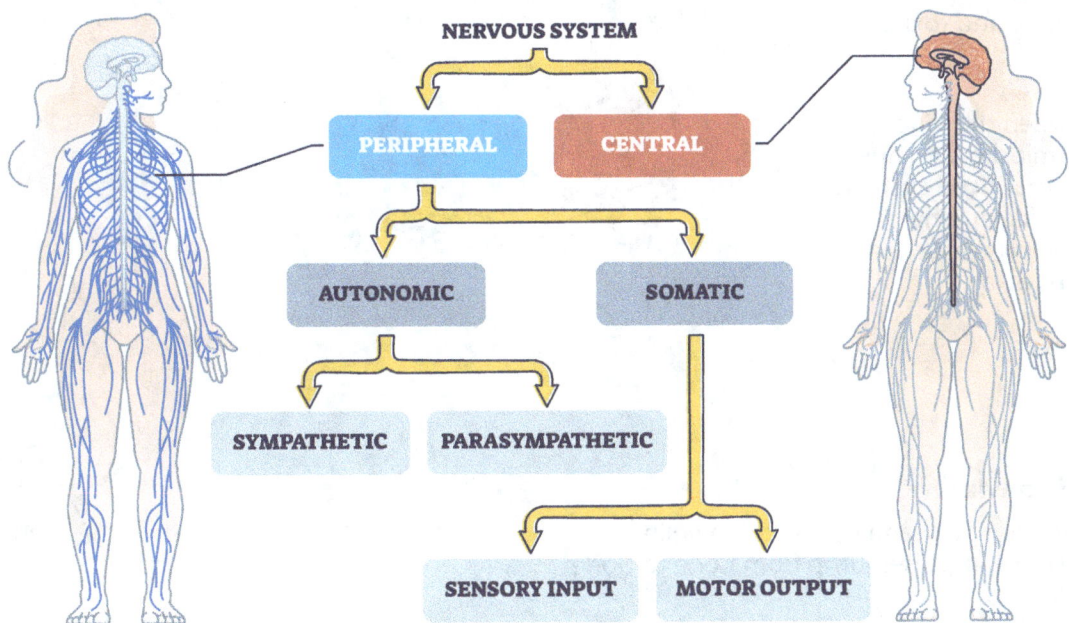

101

The brain

Cerebral cortex
Outer layer of the brain. Where thinking, memory, language and decision making occur.

Hypothalamus
Link between brain and endocrine system. It regulates homeostasis e.g. body temperature.

Cerebellum
Responsible for balance and posture.

Pituitary gland
Produces hormones e.g. ADH.

Brain stem
Connects brain to spinal cord. Manages basic functions which keep you alive like breathing.

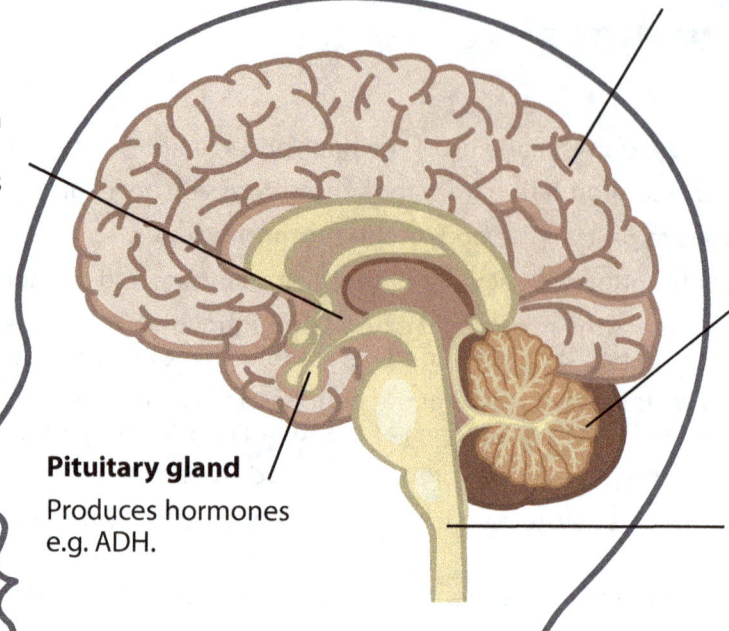

The **meninges** are three membranes which cover the brain and spinal cord and protects them from physical damage and toxins.

Between the innermost and middle meninges, **cerebral fluid** cushions the brain and helps transport waste and toxins away.

Bone — Dura mater
Brain — Arachnoid
— Pia mater
Meninges

Neurones

Node of Ranvier
Gaps between Schwann cells in the myelin sheath. Nerve impulses jump from node to node.

Dendrite
Connect to other neurones with synapses

Synaptic nob
End of axon. Releases neurotransmitters to communicate with other cells.

Axon
Long part of neurone. Nerve impulses travel away from the soma down the axon.

Nucleus
Controls the neurone

Myelin sheath
Covers most of the axon to speed up the nerve impulses along the axon.

Schwann cell
Cell that the myelin sheath is made of. Wraps around the axon.

Soma
Cell body of the neurone

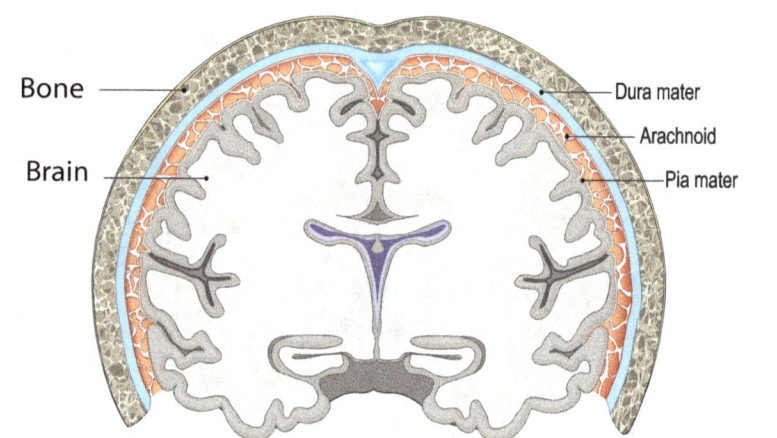

Nerve action

A nerve impulse is also known as an **action potential**. An action potential is when a change in electrical charge travels down the neurone.

- In the resting state, the outside of the axon is slightly **positive** and the inside slightly negative.
- When an action potential is triggered this difference in charge flips so the outside is **negative**. This change travels quickly along the neurone.

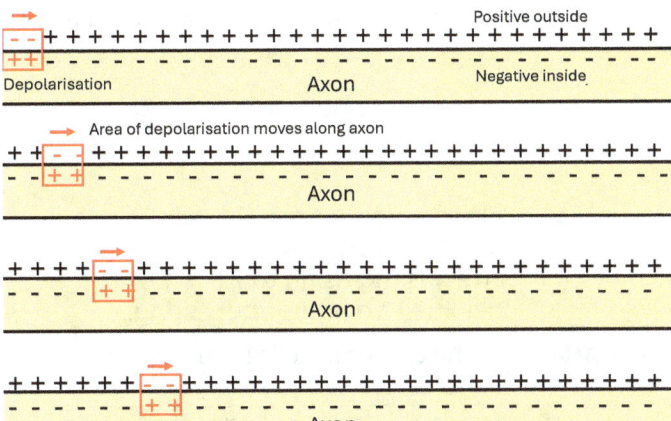

An action potential

Synapse

A synapse is a small gap between one nerve and the next. Signals must travel across a synapse using **neurotransmitters** which are special chemicals.

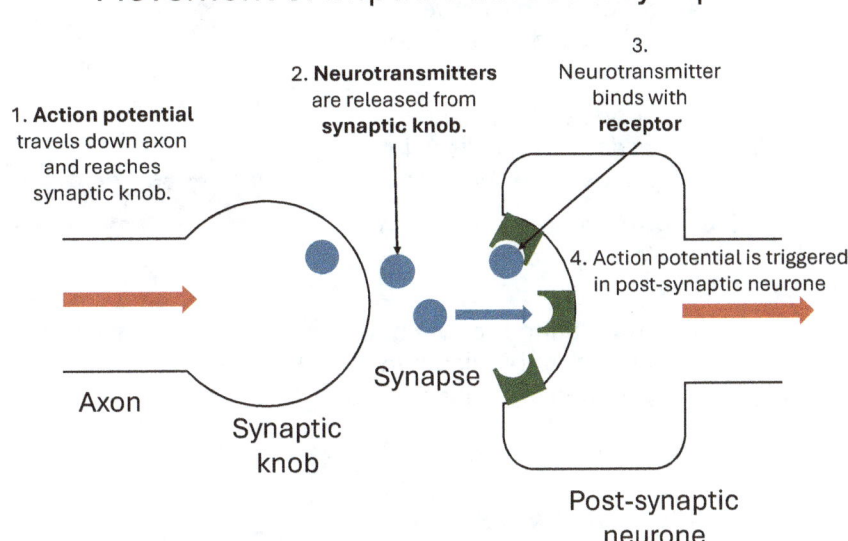

Movement of impulse across a synapse

5.2 Homeostasis

- **Homeostasis** is the process by which the body is kept in a stable condition despite changes outside and inside the body.
- The processes in the body work best if conditions are stable.

Homeostasis involves:

- A **variable** – something which might change such as body temperature, blood glucose levels or fluid levels.
- **Receptors** – sense cells which constantly monitor the level of the variable and send this information to the control centre.
- **Control centre** – area of the brain which controls this aspect of homeostasis such as the hypothalamus which controls body temperature.
- **Effectors** – glands or muscles which are stimulated by the control centre to take action to bring the level of the variable back to normal.
- **Negative feedback mechanism** – process of receptors detecting changes, informing the control centre which stimulates effectors to bring the variable to normal levels. When the variable is at its normal level the homeostatic mechanism will stop.

Homeostatic mechanisms

Specific set of receptors, control centre and effectors that maintain something specific at stable levels.

Control of regulation and blood glucose

Variable	Blood glucose normal level – between 4 and 5.4 mmol per litre after fasting rising to 7.8 mmol per litre two hours after eating.
Receptors	Alpha and beta cells in the pancreas.
Control centre	The alpha and beta cells act as a control centre for blood glucose control.
Effectors	**Insulin** – a hormone which lowers glucose after eating by: » Stimulating the liver and muscles to store glucose as glycogen. » Bonds with insulin receptors on cells to let glucose into the cells. **Glucagon** – a hormone which raises blood glucose when levels are low by: » Stimulating the liver and muscles to break down glycogen into glucose.

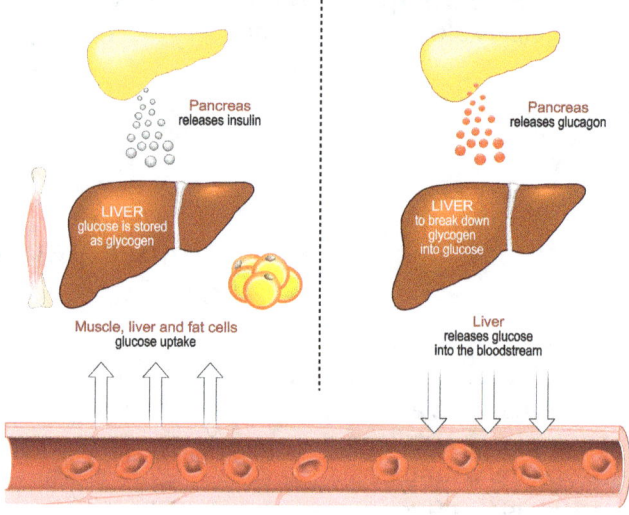

Control and regulation of water levels

Variable	Body fluid levels.
Receptors	Osmoreceptors in the hypothalamus in the brain.
Control centre	The hypothalamus in the brain.
Effectors	**Antidiuretic hormone (ADH)** – released from pituitary gland when levels of water are low. Stimulates the kidneys to retain water so it is not lost as urine. **Kidney** – tubules in the kidney can reabsorb water when fluid levels are low or filter out water from the blood to make urine when fluid levels are high. Urine is stored in the bladder until it is convenient to empty the bladder.

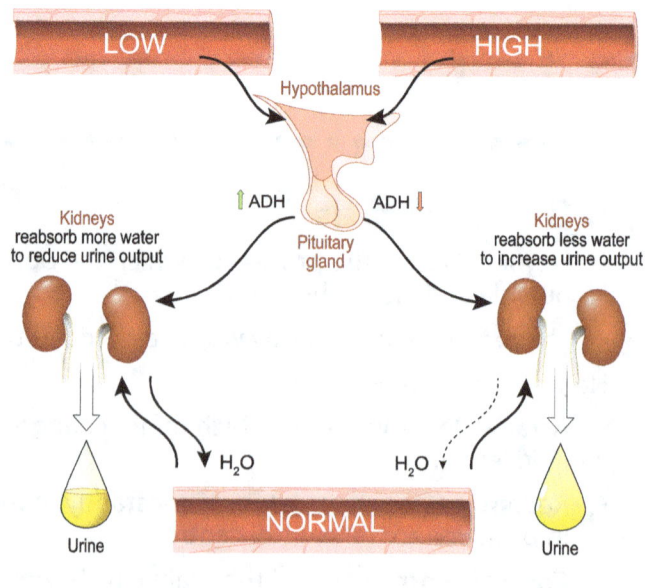

Control and regulation of body temperature

Variable	Body temperature – normally between 36.5°C and 37.5°C.
Receptors	Thermoreceptors in the skin, deep organs and hypothalamus.
Control centre	Hypothalamus in the brain.
Effectors	**Capillaries** – can let more or less blood to the surface of the skin. More blood flows to the skin surface when you are hot so heat can be lost. **Muscles** – move rapidly (shiver) when cold to generate heat. **Hair** – stands upright when cold to trap air to act as an insulate and prevent heat loss. **Sweat glands** – release sweat when hot. The evaporation of the sweat from the skin cools the body down.

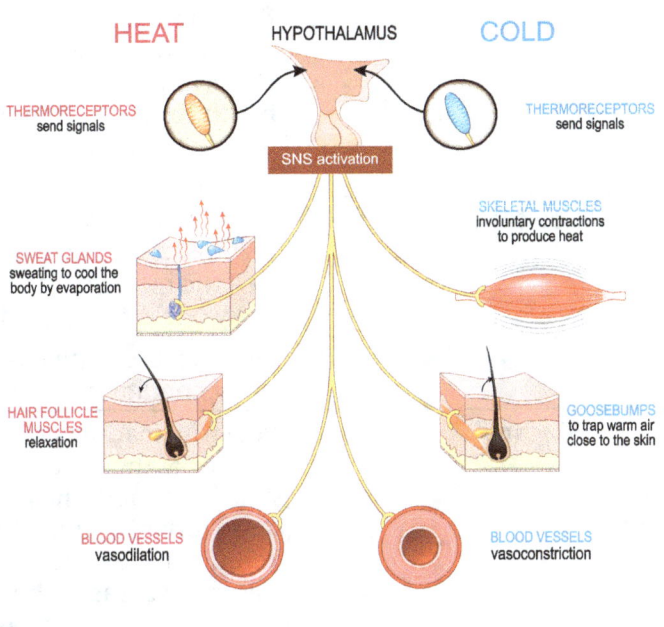

5.3 Conditions of the control of regulatory systems

Ischaemic strokes

Causes

Ischaemic strokes are caused by blood clots in the brain.

- The clot restricts the flow of blood in the blood vessel. Nerve cells that are supplied by that blood vessel will not get enough oxygen and nutrients and will be damaged or die.
- Different parts of the brain control different body functions. The symptoms of a stroke depend on where in the brain the damage is.

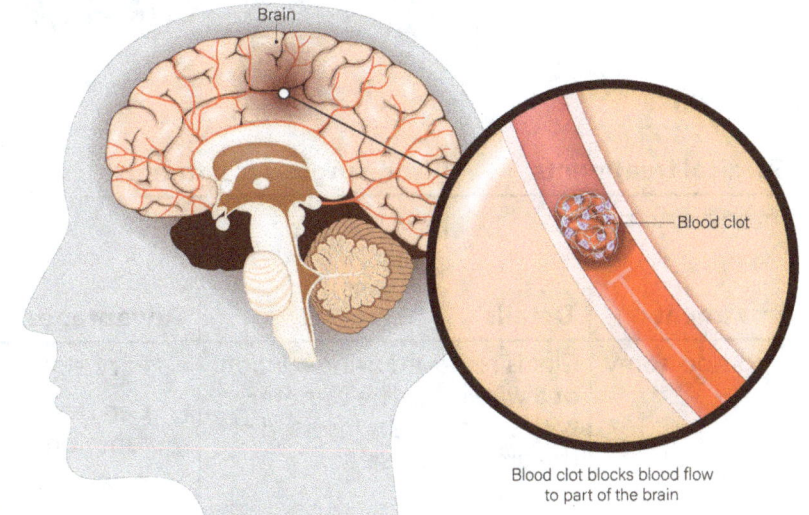

Blood clot blocks blood flow to part of the brain

Signs and symptoms

- Dropping of the face on one side as the part of the brain that controls those face muscles are damaged.
- Weakness in the arms due to damage to the parts of the brain controlling the arm muscles.
- Slurred speech due to damage to speech areas of the brain.
- Headache.
- Blurred vision due to damage to vision areas of the brain.
- Loss of consciousness (at time of stroke).

Diagnosis and monitoring

Method	Details	How and when it is used
Physical examination	The doctor will look at the patient's face and see if they can smile. They will ask them to raise their arms to check arm movement or squeeze their hands to check strength. They will ask questions and see if the patient has slurred speech.	This will be the first stage of diagnosis and is carried out immediately that a stroke is suspected.
Blood tests	Blood tests look for high cholesterol to look for risk factors. Seeing how well the blood clots can indicate how likely one is to occur in the brain. Blood tests can be used to rule out other conditions.	Can be used to help rule out other causes. Cannot be used by themselves to confirm a stroke.
MRI scans	Powerful magnets are used to make images of the part of the body being scanned. The machine is like a large tunnel that the head is passed through to scan. It can be used to find damaged areas of the brain.	Can be used to confirm a diagnosis made by physical examination. Can be used to assess the extent of damage and decide on best treatment options. Can be used to check how well treatments have worked.

Treatments

Surgical treatments	Non-surgical treatments
Thrombectomy	Thrombolysis

Treatment	Details	Advantages	Disadvantages
Thrombectomy	Clot is removed using suction or a wire loop. The catheter with the device is inserted at the groin or wrist.	• Very effective. • Can retain brain functions. • Only small cuts to the wrist or groin reduces risk of complications.	• Must be carried out within a few hours to be effective. • There is a small chance of infections. • Clot may be difficult to reach making it unsuitable.
Thrombolysis	Strong medication is given to dissolve the clot. This restores blood flow.	• Can be added to an intravenous drip making it quick and easy to carry out. • Fewer risks than surgery. • Good at removing small clots.	• Must be carried out within a few hours to be effective. • Increased risk of bleeding due to inability of blood to clot. • Not suitable for people with blood clotting problems.

Factors making strokes more likely

- **Obesity** increases the risk of stroke as it increases atherosclerosis (see cardiovascular system). It also increases risk of high blood pressure which damages blood vessels making clots more likely.
- **Diets** high in salt increase blood pressure. Low fibre diets increase plaque formation.
- **Smoking** puts harmful chemicals into the blood which increase the risk of clots. Damage to the brain will be worse in smokers as their blood can carry less oxygen.
- **Diabetes** increases the risk of atherosclerosis which causes plaque to form. People with diabetes have blood which clots more easily.
- **Stress** increases blood pressure. It also makes unhealthy lifestyle choices such as smoking, drinking and overeating more likely.
- **Hypertension** is when the blood pressure is permanently higher than it should be. It damages the blood vessels and encourages clots to form.

Control and prevention

Medication	Lifestyle changes
Statins – lower cholesterol reducing risk of clots. **Anti-coagulants** – make it harder for the blood to clot so that it is less likely a clot will form in the brain. **Beta blockers** – lower blood pressure which is a major cause of ischaemic strokes.	**Losing weight** – reduces blood pressure and cholesterol levels making clots less likely. **Reducing fat and salt in diet** – Also reduces blood pressure and cholesterol levels. **Stopping smoking** – stops the harmful chemicals that damage blood vessels, reduces risk of clots forming. **Reducing stress** – lowers blood pressure. **Regular exercise** – lowers blood pressure, improves blood circulation, helps maintain a healthy weight.

Impact of strokes on the individual

Physical	Intellectual
- Weakness down one side effects mobility and ability to do day-to-day tasks. - Can affect vision. - Can cause fatigue. - Can cause speech difficulties.	- Can affect memory. - It can be harder to think clearly. - It will be harder to take part in activities which are intellectually stimulating. - Fatigue makes it harder to concentrate.
Emotional	**Social**
- Difficulty coming to terms with changes to life the stroke has caused. - Anxiety about coping or about further strokes. - Stroke damage can directly affect a person's mood or their ability to control their mood. - Stroke damage can lead to personality changes.	- Harder to communicate as both understanding and being able to speak can be affected – aphasia. - It is harder to socialise with people if you are physically disabled. - The individual may have had to give up work due to the stroke, so they miss out on social contact they got at work.

Type 2 diabetes

Cells in the body need **glucose** to make energy. The body derives glucose from carbohydrates.

Cells need to get the right amount of glucose. Glucose levels in the blood are controlled by the hormones **insulin** and glucagon.

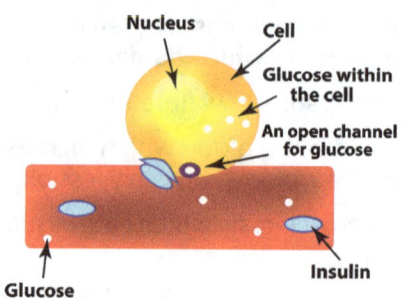

Normal

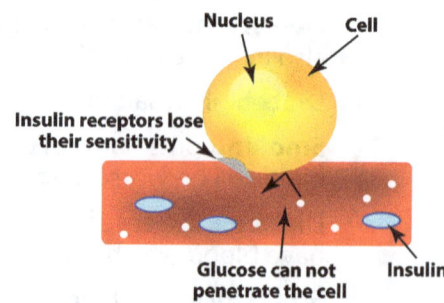

Type 2 diabetes

- **Insulin** lowers blood glucose levels and gets glucose into cells where it is used to make energy.
- **Type 2 diabetes** affects insulin production and how the body responds to it.

Causes

- Insulin receptors on the surface of the cells stop working so insulin can no longer get into cells. This keeps blood glucose levels high and prevents glucose getting into the cells, so it cannot be used for energy.
- When insulin receptors are not working properly it is known as **insulin resistance**.
- The pancreas can also become damaged, often due to being overweight, and reduces or stops its production of insulin.

Signs and symptoms

- **Fatigue** – because glucose cannot be used to make energy in the cells.
- **Unexplained weight loss** – because fats and proteins are used to make energy instead.
- **Thirst** – because glucose is removed in the urine, so a lot of urine is passed which needs to be replaced by drinking.
- **Increased urination** – glucose leaves the body as urine in the kidneys. High glucose concentrations in the urine draw water to it by osmosis so more water is lost in the urine.

Diagnosis and monitoring

Method	Details	How and when it is used
Blood glucose test	Glucose levels of 7 mmol per litre or higher after an 8-hour fast indicates diabetes. Other blood tests see how quickly blood glucose is lowered after a meal.	Blood tests are used to confirm the diagnosis. They are also used to monitor blood glucose every day to ensure the condition is being managed properly.
Urine test	Detect the presence of glucose in the urine. People without diabetes do not have glucose in their urine.	A quick test which can be used as an indication before a blood test is carried out.
Eye test	A dye is injected into the blood vessels of the eye before the retina is photographed. This shows areas of damage to the retina known as diabetic retinopathy which is caused by diabetes.	This test is not used to diagnose diabetes. It is used to detect damage to the eye caused by diabetes.
Neuropathy test	This test looks for numbness, slow reflexes and muscle weakness. These are caused by damage to nerves caused by the diabetes.	This test is not used to diagnose diabetes but to monitor whether the condition is damaging the nerves.

Treatments

Surgical treatments	Non-surgical treatments	Lifestyle changes
Gastric banding	Metformin	Lose weight

Treatment	How it works
Gastric band	• During an operation, a band is put around part of the stomach to reduce its size, so the patient loses weight. Being overweight is the main cause of type 2 diabetes. Losing weight can put a person into remission.
Metformin	• Taken as a tablet, this medication makes the body more sensitive to insulin, so it reduces insulin resistance. It also reduces the amount of glucose that is made in the liver from glycogen.
Losing weight	• Reduces the symptoms and can put the person into remission. Being overweight increases insulin sensitivity and causes fat build-up in the pancreas which stops it from making insulin.

Treatment	Advantages	Disadvantages
Gastric band	• Very effective in causing weight loss. • Causes a reduction in insulin resistance so individual can reduce their reliance on medication. • Helps the patient manage blood glucose levels so they are less likely to suffer from the complications of diabetes.	• Many people do not meet the strict criteria for the surgery. • It dramatically changes what a person can eat and how much. Many people struggle to adjust to this change. • It is a major operation with risks which include infection and damage to the digestive system.
Metformin	• It is effective at managing blood glucose levels. • Easy to administer and does not require invasive surgery. • It also reduces the risk of heart attacks and strokes which are more common in people with type 2 diabetes.	• Can give side effects of nausea and diarrhoea. • Not suitable for people with heart failure or kidney disease. • Does not work for everyone.
Losing weight	• Reduces insulin resistance so the individual's insulin will work better. • There will be less need for other treatments like metformin. • It will improve overall health, give them more energy and make it less likely they will suffer from other disorders.	• It can be very difficult to lose weight. • Changes to the lifestyle need to be permanent – a temporary diet is not enough. • It can take a long time to lose enough weight.

5: Control and regulatory systems

Factors making type 2 diabetes more likely

- **Obesity** can cause the pancreas to produce less insulin and increases insulin resistance.
- Being **45 years old or older** increases the risk as we produce less insulin as we get older. We also lose muscle mass which is used to store excess glucose as glycogen.
- **Inactivity** makes weight gain more likely. Not using muscles means that energy from glucose is not used as much so glucose builds up in the blood.
- **Ethnicity** has an impact as some ethnic groups are more prone to the disease than others. This includes people of African descent, people of South Asian descent, people of Central and Southern American, descent, and people of native American descent.

Control and prevention

Method	How it works
Lose weight	Reduces insulin resistance and enables to pancreas to make more insulin.
Dietary changes	Improves overall health and reduces the amount of high glucose foods (carbohydrates) that are eaten. Diet should include plenty of fruit and vegetables, food with a low glycaemic index, eating regularly, limiting sugary food and drinks, drinking plenty of fluids and eating plenty of fibre.
Regular exercise	Helps control body weight, uses up more glucose so it is less likely to build up in the blood and it improves overall health.

Impact of diabetes on the individual

Physical	Intellectual
- Lack of energy. - Need to go to the toilet frequently. - May have problems with vision, known as **diabetic retinopathy**. - Wounds take longer to heal. - Increased risk of heart disease, kidney disease, strokes, circulatory problems.	- Difficulty concentrating due to lack of energy.
Emotional	**Social**
- Anxiety about complications and keeping blood sugar levels down. - Lifestyle changes may be difficult to come to terms with.	- Regular appointments may interrupt social life. - Changes in diet may make it harder to go out with others for a meal. - More likely to become socially isolated.

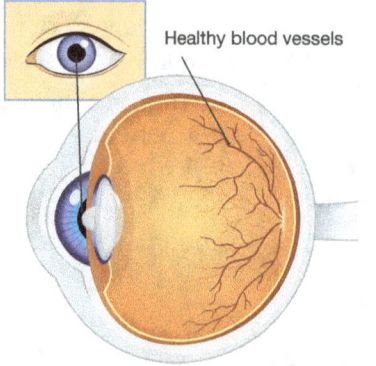

Normal Eye

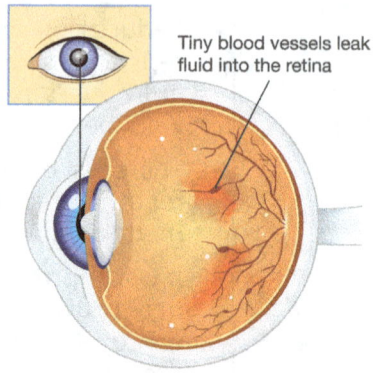

Eye with Retinopathy

Study Tips!

- You need to know where each of the components listed in the specification are located and what each does.
- You may need to be able to label diagrams of the brain and of both sensory and motor neurones.
- Remember that neurotransmitters use the normal rules of diffusion in that they diffuse from areas of high concentration (at the synaptic knob) to areas of low concentration (at the post synaptic neurone).
- Remember that homeostasis is a process of keeping a certain aspect of the body stable despite external or internal changes. There are many factors that are kept stable due to homeostasis – you need to be clear about which you are talking about e.g. homeostasis of body temperature or homeostasis of blood glucose levels.
- You can think of a negative feedback mechanism as switching between measures to bring something back to normal levels. This switching will only happen when levels have returned to normal.

Important terms!

Nerve impulse – Also known as an action potential, a nerve impulse is the method used for messages to travel along a neurone. It is caused by a difference of charge across the neurone membrane. During a nerve impulse the charge flips and this change in charge travels down the neurone.

Mmol per litre – Stands for millimoles per litre and is a measure of the concentration of glucose in blood when measuring blood glucose levels.

Osmoreceptor – Sensory receptor or sense cell within the body which can detect changes in fluid levels in the body.

Thermoreceptor – Sensory receptor or cell which can detect changes in temperature within the body.

Cholesterol – A type of steroid which is a biological molecule made mostly of fat. Cholesterol plays an important part in the workings of the body including being part of cell membranes. However, too much can cause problems with the cardiovascular system.

Aphasia – Where is speech or language understanding is affected by damage to the areas of the brain which control speech. The exact effects depend on the exact area damaged.

Osmosis – Movement of water from one area to another through a selectively permeable membrane (lets some substances through but not others) from an area of high water concentration to an area of low water concentration.

Diabetic retinopathy – Damage caused to the retina due to diabetes. It is caused by high blood glucose levels which damage the blood vessels in the retina and, if not controlled, can lead to loss of sight.

Remission – A period when the signs and symptoms of a disease reduce or disappear altogether. It does not necessarily mean that the disease is cured. The symptoms may come back.

Glycaemic index – A scale between 0 and 100 used to rank how quickly carbohydrates in a particular type of food raise blood glucose levels. For example, white bread has a GI of 75 which means it raises blood glucose quickly. Whereas chickpeas have a much lower GI of 28.

5: Control and regulatory systems

Recap Questions

1. What is the function of the central nervous system?
2. What does the autonomic nervous system control?
3. What is a sensory neurone?
4. What is the function of the hypothalamus?
5. Where in the brain are the meninges?
6. Where would you find a Schwann cell?
7. What role does a neurotransmitter play in nerve action?
8. What is the role of antidiuretic hormone in the regulation of water in the body?
9. What is the difference between insulin and glucagon?
10. What are the effectors when the body gets too cold?
11. What is the cause of an ischaemic stroke?
12. Why might someone suffering an ischaemic stroke have slurred speech?
13. What is thrombolysis?
14. How can beta blockers help to reduce the risk of ischaemic strokes?
15. Give two symptoms of type 2 diabetes.
16. What role can metformin play in treating type 2 diabetes?
17. Why can regular exercise help prevent type 2 diabetes?

Revision Quiz

1. What does the QRS wave in an ECG show?
2. How can a healthy diet help relieve the symptoms of endometriosis?
3. Where is the bicuspid valve located in the heart?
4. What is the role of luteinising hormone?
5. What is the epiglottis?
6. Why is someone who uses vibrating tools at greater risk of carpal tunnel syndrome?
7. What hormone changes lead to menopause?
8. Give two symptoms of bowel polyps.
9. What are the links between stress and angina?
10. Where in the cell does anaerobic respiration occur?
11. What is an anti-coagulant?
12. What is the role of the vagina in reproduction?
13. Name a physical impact of pneumonia on an individual.
14. What are villi and what do they do?
15. What role does inflammation play in osteoarthritis?
16. When does menopause usually occur?
17. What is joint fusing?

Assessment practice

1. Which part of the brain is responsible for posture, balance and movement? (1)

2. Fill in the gaps: The brain is protected by three _____ which are membranes which cover the surface of the brain and spinal cord. The _____ is located between two of the membranes. (2)

3. What transports a signal from one neurone to the next across a synapse? (1)

4. Which is **incorrect** about transmission of signals across a synapse? (1)

   A Neurotransmitters diffuse across the synapse from the synaptic knob.

   B Neurotransmitters bind with receptors on the post-synaptic neurone.

   C Neurotransmitters can trigger another nerve or a muscle.

   D Neurotransmitters are made in the synaptic knob when the nerve impulse reaches it.

5. What is detected by receptors as part of the homeostatic process? (1)

6. Where in the brain are control centres related to homeostasis located? (1)

7. State two hormones involved in blood glucose homeostasis. (2)

8. Which of the following is **incorrect** about blood glucose homeostasis? (1)

   A Glucagon causes glycogen to be broken down into glucose.

   B Insulin is released shortly after eating food.

   C The cells need insulin to break down glucose to produce energy.

   D Glucagon is released if the individual has not eaten for a while.

9. Where is the control centre for the control of water levels? (1)

10. What effect does ADH have on whether water is retained in the body or lost as urine? (1)

11. State three effectors for cooling the body down if too hot. (3)

12. What type of neurone sends messages from the brain to the sweat glands? (1)

13. What will a doctor look for during a physical examination to diagnose a stroke? (2)

14. What is the name of the procedure by which a clot is removed by suction or a wire loop? (2)

15. Fill in the gaps: Diets that are high in _____ and _____ make ischaemic strokes more likely to occur. Whereas diets high in _____ make them less likely to occur. (3)

16. Which is **not true** about the use of blood tests to diagnose diabetes? (1)

    A They can detect if blood glucose levels are not in the normal range.

    B They can be used to see how quickly the body can deal with sugar that has been eaten.

    C They can be used to monitor treatments by keeping a record of readings throughout the day.

    D They can be used to measure glucagon levels.

17. State the name of the medication which reduces insulin resistance. (1)

18. Explain the role of the meninges. (4)

19. Explain the role of antidiuretic hormone (ADH). (4)

20. Explain how homeostasis maintains body temperature when the body is surrounded by cold conditions. (4)

21. Describe how ischaemic strokes are diagnosed. (6)

22. Explain why smoking increases the risk of ischaemic strokes. (4)

23. Discuss the benefits and limitations of treating type 2 diabetes with gastric band surgery. (6)

> Manuel (54) has just been rushed into hospital following a suspected stroke. He is overweight and has high blood pressure. The doctors at the hospital are deciding which treatment is best for him. They are considering either a thrombectomy or thrombolysis.
>
> 24. Discuss the benefits and limitations of each treatment and form a judgement as to which treatment would suit Manuel best. (9)

6: Reproductive system

Female reproductive system

Structure and function of the female reproductive system

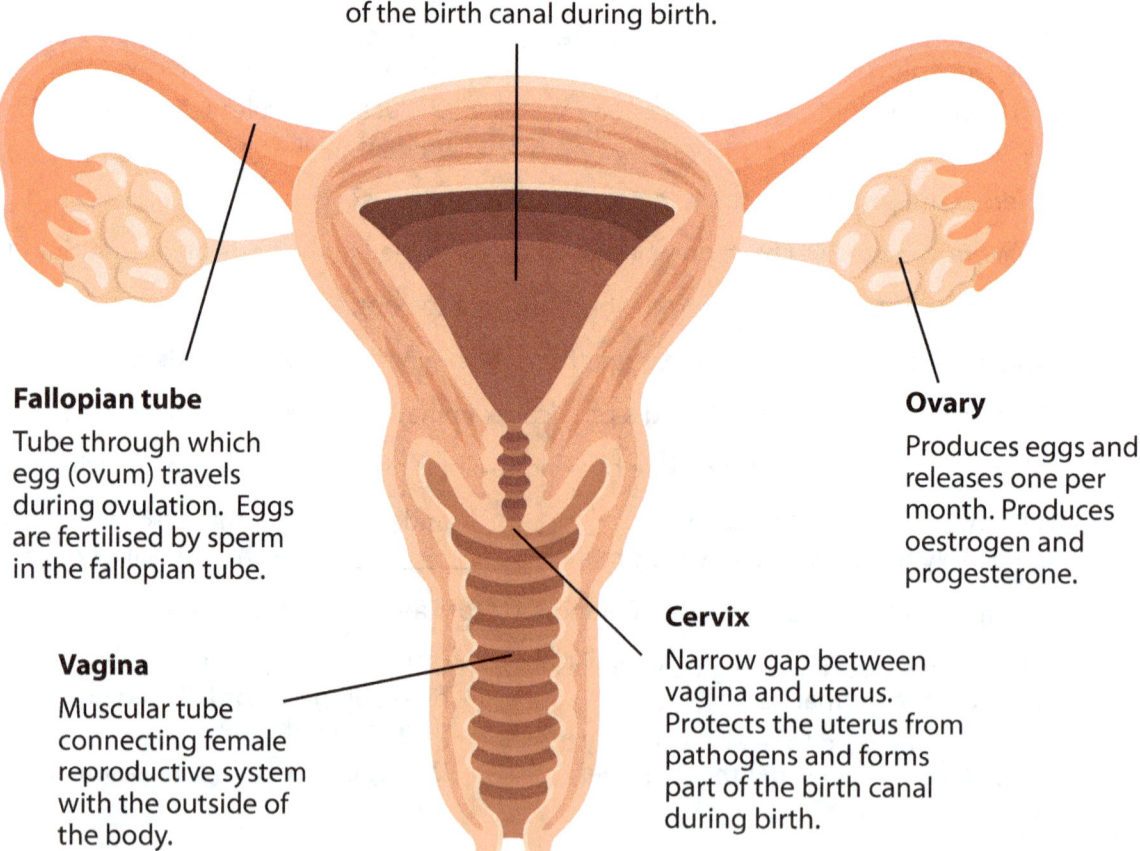

Uterus
Muscular sac which nourishes the baby during pregnancy. Forms part of the birth canal during birth.

Fallopian tube
Tube through which egg (ovum) travels during ovulation. Eggs are fertilised by sperm in the fallopian tube.

Vagina
Muscular tube connecting female reproductive system with the outside of the body.

Cervix
Narrow gap between vagina and uterus. Protects the uterus from pathogens and forms part of the birth canal during birth.

Ovary
Produces eggs and releases one per month. Produces oestrogen and progesterone.

Menstrual cycle

The menstrual cycle is about 28 days long.

- It is the cycle of shedding and thickening of the **endometrium** and ovulation in the middle of the cycle.
- It is controlled by four different hormones: FSH, oestrogen, LH and progesterone.
  » **Follicle-stimulating hormone** (FSH) stimulates follicles to develop.

» **Oestrogen** causes the endometrium to thicken.

» **Luteinising hormone** (LH) stimulates ovulation.

» **Progesterone** maintains the endometrium to prepare for pregnancy.

There are four stages of the menstrual cycle as show in the table overleaf.

Stage	Duration	What happens?	Hormone levels
Menstruation	From day 1-5	The endometrium is shed – having a period.	Low levels of both oestrogen and progesterone.
Follicular phase	From day 1 - 13	Follicles develop. One becomes dominant and will release its egg during ovulation. The endometrium begins to thicken again.	Controlled by FSH which is at high levels. Oestrogen gradually increases during this phase.
Ovulation	On about day 14	An egg (ovum) is released from the ovary.	Triggered by a sudden spike in LH levels.
Luteal phase	Day 15 - 28	Follicle becomes the corpus luteum which secretes oestrogen and progesterone. The endometrium lining thickens. However, if pregnancy has not occurred by the end of the cycle, the corpus luteum breaks down stimulating the beginning of the next cycle.	Oestrogen and progesterone levels remain high during this phase until the end when there is a sudden drop due to the break down of the corpus luteum.

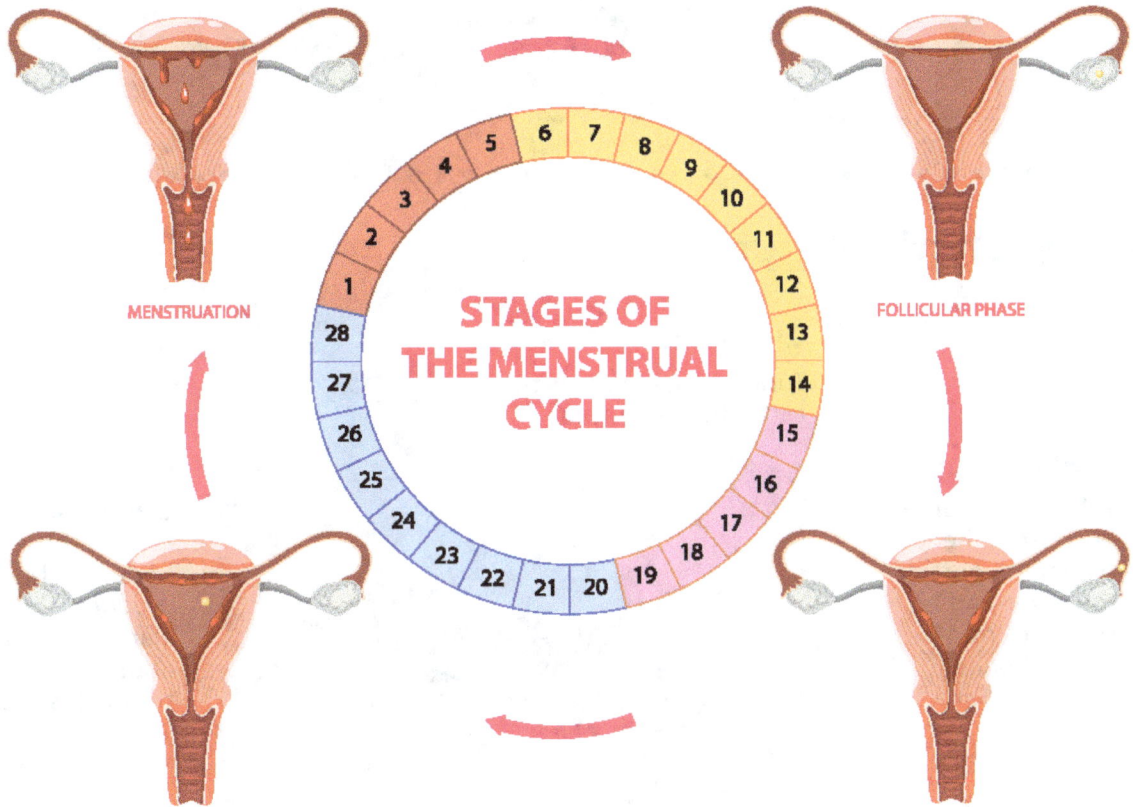

Menopause

Menopause is the end of the fertile period of a woman's life. Menopause is defined as happening when the individual has not had a period for 12 months.

- It is caused by a reduction in both oestrogen and progesterone.
- The menstrual cycle stops.
- The individual will no longer have periods.
- The individual will not be able to get pregnant.
- Menopause usually happens between the ages of 45 and 55.
- Before menopause is a period of hormone changes and unpleasant symptoms known as **perimenopause**.

Symptoms of menopause

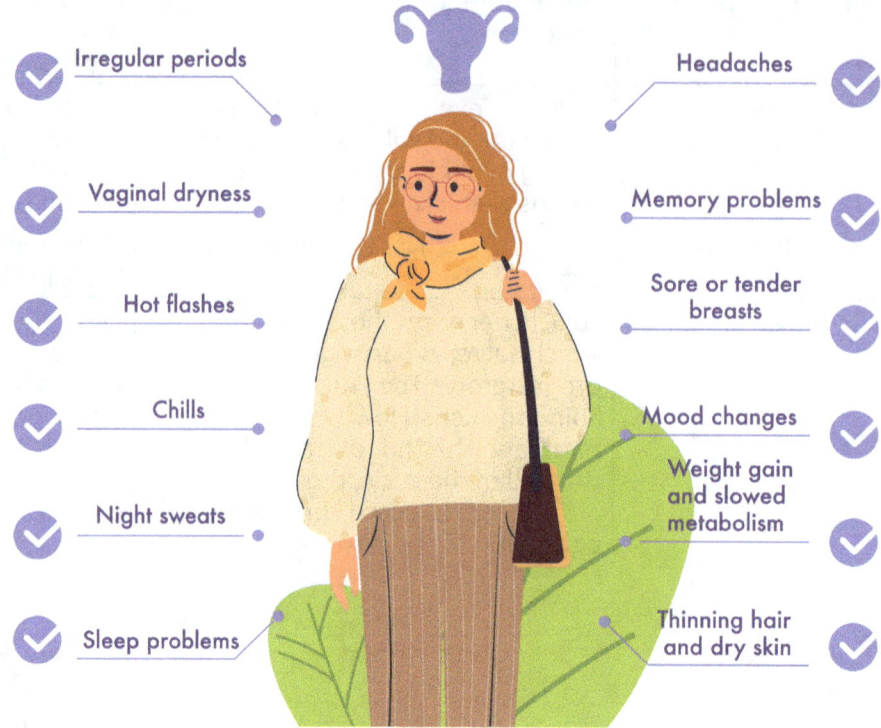

- Irregular periods
- Vaginal dryness
- Hot flashes
- Chills
- Night sweats
- Sleep problems
- Headaches
- Memory problems
- Sore or tender breasts
- Mood changes
- Weight gain and slowed metabolism
- Thinning hair and dry skin

Male reproductive system

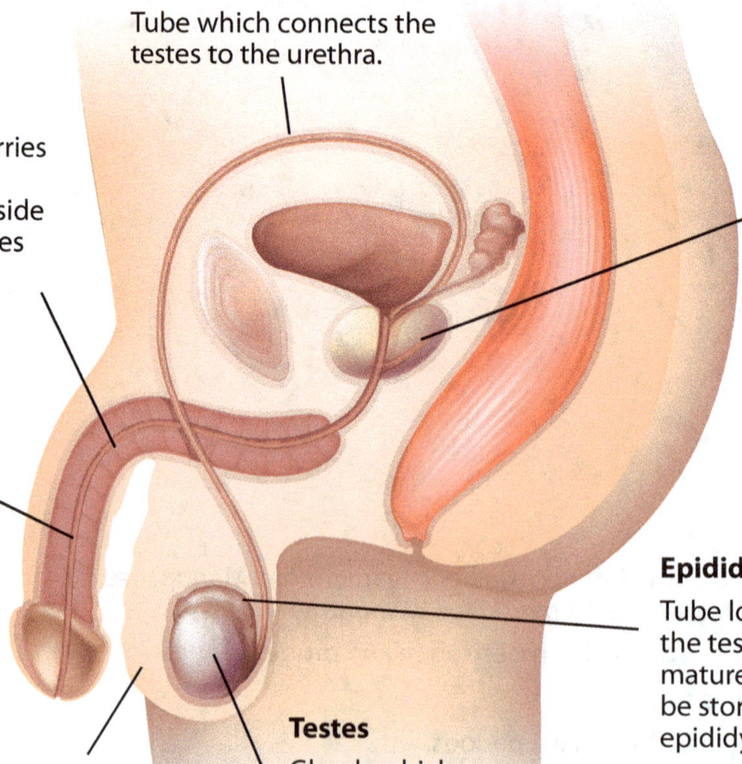

Vas deferens
Tube which connects the testes to the urethra.

Urethra
Tube which carries urine from the bladder to outside the body. Carries semen during ejaculation.

Prostate
Gland which wraps around the urethra under the bladder. It produces fluid during ejaculation which nourishes the sperm and stimulates them to swim.

Penis
Contains erectile tissue to allow it to enter the vagina and release sperm by the cervix.

Epididymis
Tube located behind the testis. Sperm mature and can be stored in the epididymis.

Scrotum
Skin which holds the testes in place outside the body. Helps control the temperature of the testes which need to be below body temperature to produce sperm.

Testes
Glands which produce sperm and the hormone testosterone.

6.2 Conditions of the reproductive system

Endometriosis

Endometriosis is when endometrial tissue grows in other parts of the body than the uterus.

Endometriosis often affects the **ovaries**, **fallopian tubes**, and the **pelvic region** in general. Endometriosis tissue thickens and is then shed with the menstrual cycle just as the lining of the uterus thickens and then is shed. The blood cannot always escape from the body so builds up and causes pain and swelling. There can also be tissue damage in the area which causes scarring.

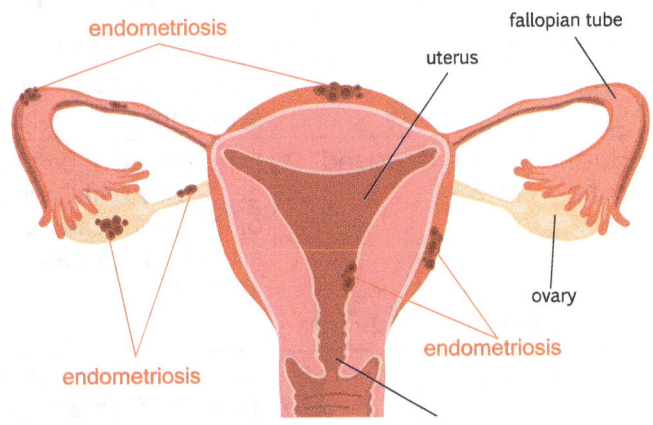

Signs and symptoms

- Pelvic pain.
- Pain during or after sex.
- Heavy periods.
- Severe period pains.
- Difficulties conceiving.

Diagnosis and monitoring

Method	Details	How and when it is used
Pelvic examination	The doctor will feel for cysts and nodules in the abdomen which can be caused by endometriosis. They will press on the abdomen to see where the pain is.	Carried out by the doctor to narrow down the options when the individual complains of the symptoms.
MRI scan	Strong magnets are used to create an image of the part of the body affected. Areas affected by endometriosis will show up.	Useful when planning surgery as it will show where the surgery is needed.
Ultrasound	High frequency sound is passed through the body and used to make images of the body. Can include both external and internal examinations.	It cannot find endometriosis tissue but can find cysts and nodules which are caused by the condition.
Laparoscopy	A camera (laparoscope) is inserted into the abdominal cavity under general anaesthetic. Areas of endometriosis can be seen and can be removed.	Used to diagnose the condition but surgery can be done to remove the tissue at the same time.

Treatments

Surgical treatments	Non-surgical treatments
Laparoscopic removal of endometriosis tissue	Pain relief
Hysterectomy	Hormonal medicines and contraceptives

Treatment	How it works
Laparoscopic removal of endometriosis tissue	A laparoscope is used to find the endometriosis tissue which can be burned out using lasers or cut out.
Hysterectomy	A hysterectomy is major surgery to remove the uterus and ovaries.
Pain relief	Medication like paracetamol or ibuprofen can be used to ease the symptoms.
Hormonal medicines and contraceptives	Hormones can be taken to prevent the endometriosis tissue from getting too thick which will reduce the pain. The contraceptive pill or injections can be used or hormone medication to put someone in artificial menopause.

Treatment	Advantages	Disadvantages
Laparoscopic removal of endometriosis tissue	• Small cuts needed make it less invasive than other types of surgery. • It can be done at the same time as a laparoscopy used to diagnose the condition. • It is effective in reducing pain. • It does not prevent the individual from getting pregnant.	• It does not relieve symptoms for everyone. • Sometimes the endometriosis tissue can come back. • Surgery increases the risk of infections. • Some people react badly to anaesthetic. • Surgery can lead to heavy bleeding.
Hysterectomy	• Usually effective in relieving the pain. • The individual will no longer have periods. • Contraception will no longer be needed as the individual will not be able to get pregnant.	• Major surgery can take a while to recover from. • Removal of the ovaries stimulates early menopause which comes with health risks of its own. • The surgery cannot be reversed so it will not be possible to have a baby. • There may still be pain if the endometriosis tissue is somewhere else in the body.
Pain relief	• Pain killers are easy to get, and you don't need a prescription. • They work quickly to relieve pain.	• Many people find that they are not strong enough. • Long-term use of medication can cause problems like ulcers.
Hormonal medicines and contraceptives	• Can be very effective in reducing pain. • Slows the progress of the disease and reduces the amount of scarring that will occur. • There are a range of different types of treatment to choose from.	• It does not cure the condition. • The hormones which induce artificial menopause increase the risk of conditions like osteoporosis. • It is not possible to get pregnant while taking the treatment. • There can be side effects.

Laprascopic surgery

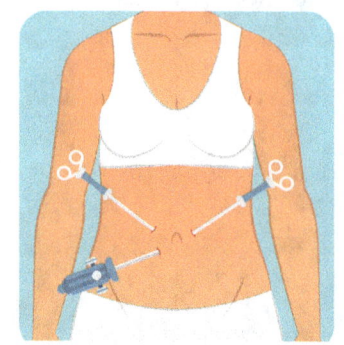
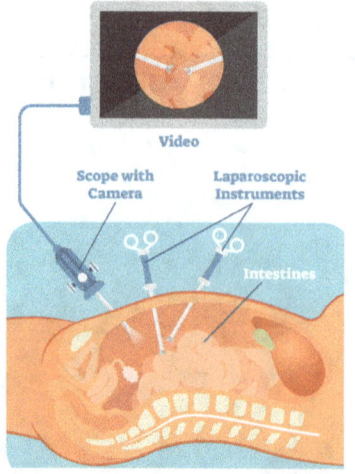

Factors making endometriosis more likely

- Having a **family history** of the disease increases the likelihood of developing endometriosis.
- **Starting periods early** (before 11 years old) also increases the risk. This could be due to longer exposure to menstrual blood.
- Having **short menstrual cycles** (of 27 days or fewer) means that the individual is having more periods and so they have more exposure to menstrual blood.
- **Heavy menstrual periods** increase the amount of contact with menstrual blood.

Control and prevention

Method	How it works
Pain relief	Pain relief does not prevent or treat the condition but eases the symptoms so the individual can get on with their life.
Hormonal medicines and contraceptives	Hormone treatment reduces the amount of bleeding during periods. Lighter periods tend to produce less pain and reduces exposure to menstrual blood which can damage tissues and cause scarring and cysts. Hormones can also shrink cysts that have already formed.
Lifestyle changes:	Lifestyle changes listed below can reduce the risk of the disease and reduce the impact for those that have the disease. Lifestyle changes can reduce inflammation which helps ease the symptoms.
Reduce stress	Stress makes the symptoms worse so reducing stress will ease them.
Dietary changes	Eating plenty of fresh fruit and vegetables, whole grains and omega-3 fats helps reduce inflammation and ease symptoms.
Exercise regularly	Exercise also reduces inflammation as well as reducing levels of oestrogen making pain easier to manage.

Impact of endometriosis on the individual

Physical	Intellectual
- Pain can be severe. - Periods can be very heavy. - Heavy bleeding may mean they do not have enough red blood cells so not enough oxygen leading to fatigue. - May have difficulty getting pregnant.	- May need to miss school or work affecting intellectual development. - Difficulty concentrating when in pain or worrying about a heavy period.
Emotional	**Social**
- Pain and anxiety can affect mental health. - Difficulty getting pregnant may be devastating for some people.	- It is harder to socialise when you are in pain. - They may avoid social interaction when having a heavy period. - Inability to have children may put a strain on their relationships.

Testicular cancer

- **Cancer** is caused by damage to DNA which causes cells to divide uncontrollably to form a tumour.
- Testicular cancer is when cells divide uncontrollably in the testes.
- Testicular cancer usually affects germ cells.

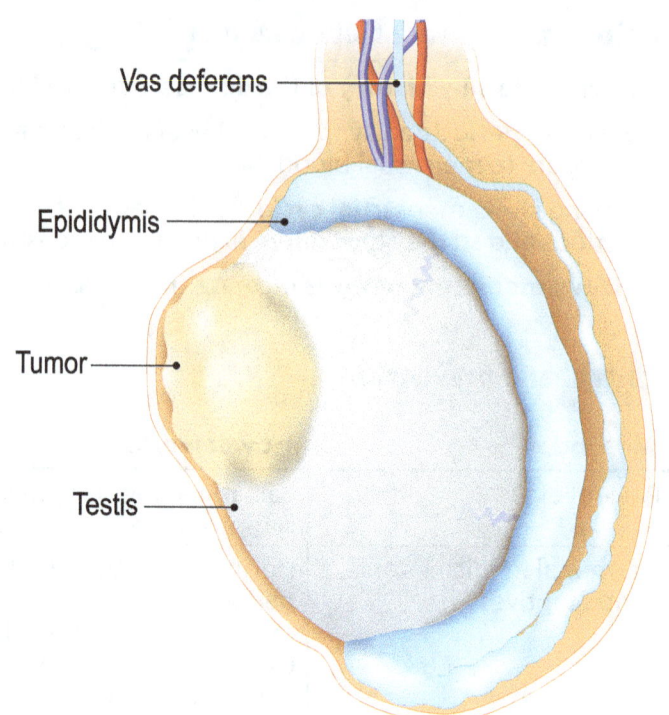

Signs and symptoms

- Lump in the testicles due to the cancerous tumour.
- Feeling of heaviness in the scrotum due to the extra tissue of the tumour.
- Pain in the testicle as the tumour presses on other tissue.
- Increased firmness in the testicle as tumours are solid masses of cells.

Diagnosis and monitoring

Method	Details	How and when it is used
Physical examination	The doctor will look at and feel the testicles to see if there are any lumps or large differences between the two.	A physical examination will take place when the individual first comes to the doctor who will send the individual for further tests.
Ultrasound	High frequency sound is used to make a picture of the testicles. It can tell the difference between a cyst and a tumour. It is possible to measure the size of the tumour.	It is used as part of the diagnosis and can be used during treatment to check the tumour is shrinking.
Blood test	Blood tests look for specific proteins known as cancer markers which indicate there is cancer in the body.	Blood tests can be done as part of the diagnosis but also regularly during treatment to monitor whether it is working.

Treatments

Surgical treatments	Non-surgical treatments
Orchidectomy	Chemotherapy

Treatment	Details	Advantages	Disadvantages
Orchidectomy	One or both testicles are removed under general anaesthetic. A prosthetic can be used so that the testicles will look and feel the same as before the surgery.	• Removes the cancer. • Quick procedure and the individual can usually go home the same day. • Tests can be done on the testicles to check the type of cancer and see if other treatments are needed.	• If both testicles are removed, the individual will not be able to have children. • Testosterone production can be reduced leading to other health problems. • Can have a big psychological impact.

Treatment	Details	Advantages	Disadvantages
Chemotherapy	Strong medication is given which kills cancer cells. It can be given as tablets or injection.	• Useful if the cancer has spread. • Removes cancer that was not removed by surgery.	• Can produce severe side effects like hair loss, nausea, vomiting, fatigue and increased likelihood of infections. • Can affect fertility

Factors making testicular cancer more likely

- **Undescended testicles** where the testicles remain in the abdominal cavity until after birth increases the risk. The risk is higher even when surgery is used to correct the undescended testicles.
- **Family history** of testicular cancer increases the risk as the individual may have a genetic predisposition.
- Being **aged between 15 and 49** increases the risk. This is probably because the cells which produce sperm are more active during this period.
- Having had **previous testicular cancer** increases the risk as the factors that increase risk will still be present.
- Having been treated with **radiotherapy** increases the risk. Radiotherapy is where radiation is used to treat cancer. Radiation affects DNA and can cause cancer.

Impact of testicular cancer on the individual

Physical	Intellectual
• Pain. • Testicles may be different sizes from each other. • Chemotherapy has unpleasant side effects. • If both testicles have been removed the individual will not be able to have children.	• Reduction in testosterone can affect concentration and memory. • Stress of the situation will also make it hard to focus on intellectual activities.
Emotional	**Social**
• Anxiety due to cancer diagnosis • Embarrassment due to the area of the body affected. • They may feel their masculinity has been affected.	• May begin to withdraw due to embarrassment. • May not be able to confide in friends about their condition. • The condition may impact on sexual health. • Low sex drive or inability to get an erection may affect intimate relationships.

Study Tips!

- Try to use the scientific name for components of the reproductive system such as ovum instead of egg and uterus instead of womb.
- It is very important to know the role that each hormone plays in controlling the menstrual cycle.
- In everyday life people often use the term 'menopause' when they mean 'perimenopause'. So if someone says they are going through the menopause they probably mean that they are going through the perimenopause and have not yet reached menopause.

> **Important terms!**
>
> **Ovulation** – The part of the menstrual cycle where a mature ovum (egg) is released from the ovary.
>
> **Follicles** – A group of cells that develop within the ovary. It contains a developing ovum. When ovulation occurs it the mature ovum is released from the follicle.
>
> **Ovum** – An ovum is the scientific name for an egg in the female reproductive system. Ova is the plural form.
>
> **Corpus luteum** – A structure which is left of the follicle after the egg has been released during ovulation. The corpus luteum secretes progesterone and some oestrogen during the luteal phase of the menstrual cycle.
>
> **Conceive** – The term used to describe the moment when the sperm fertilises the egg and begins pregnancy.
>
> **Cyst** – A lump in a body tissue. Cysts can be filled with fluid or gas or can also be solid. Most are not cancerous.
>
> **Nodule** – A solid piece of tissue which rises about the rest of the endometriosis tissue.
>
> **Laparoscope** – A medical device consisting of a flexible tube with a light and camera on one end. It can be inserted through cuts into the abdominal cavity to investigate and operate on endometriosis tissue.
>
> **Germ cell** – The type of cell which produces either ova or sperm cells.
>
> **Prosthetic** – An artificial devise that is used to replace a missing part of the body.

Recap Questions

1. Where in the female body are eggs normally fertilised by sperm?
2. What is the role of the uterus?
3. Describe what happens during the follicular phase of the menstrual cycle.
4. Name the four hormones that control the menstrual cycle.
5. What is the definition of menopause?
6. What organs do the vas deferens connect?
7. What is endometriosis?
8. Why might a doctor perform a pelvic examination to diagnose endometriosis?
9. What advantages do hormone medicines have in treating endometriosis?
10. Give two disadvantages of a hysterectomy to treat endometriosis.
11. What intellectual impacts can endometriosis have on an individual?
12. What is a germ cell?
13. What is an orchidectomy?
14. Why might a doctor perform an ultrasound to diagnose testicular cancer?
15. Why is previous radiotherapy treatment a risk factor for testicular cancer?
16. Give two social impacts on an individual of testicular cancer.
17. Name one symptom of testicular cancer.
18. Why do people who have shorter menstrual cycles have a greater risk of endometriosis?
19. Give one advantage of chemotherapy for treating testicular cancer.

Revision Quiz

1. What happens during an angioplasty?
2. What are bronchioles?
3. What is a tendon?
4. Give two adaptations of the small intestine that aid absorption of nutrients.
5. Name a common sign of DVT.
6. Why is age a risk factor for type 2 diabetes?
7. What is a pulmonary embolism?
8. Give one risk factor for carpal tunnel syndrome.
9. Name one structural adaptation of alveoli that helps with gas exchange.
10. Give two physical impacts of ischaemic strokes on an individual.
11. What is compact bone and where can you find it?
12. What is the function of a lipase enzyme?
13. Why is age a risk factor for osteoarthritis?
14. Describe the role of the pancreas in blood glucose regulation.

Assessment practice

1. Fill in the gaps: During the menstruation phase of the cycle the levels of oestrogen are _____ and the levels of progesterone are _____. (2)

2. Which is **incorrect** about the menopause? (1)

   A Levels of both oestrogen and progesterone decrease.

   B Menopause is a period of increased fertility.

   C It is defined happening after a period of 12 months without menstruation has occurred.

   D Before menopause periods become irregular.

3. Identify the structures labelled A-D on the diagram below. (4)

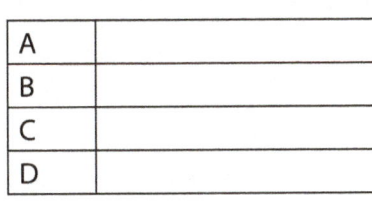
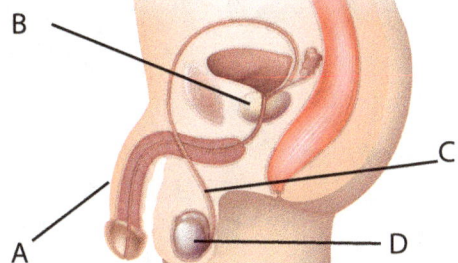

A	
B	
C	
D	

4. State the name of the gland in the male reproductive system which releases a fluid during ejaculation which stimulates the sperm to move. (1)

5. Which is **correct** about endometriosis? (1)

   A It is caused by the lining of the uterus (endometrium) becoming too thick.

   B It is not affected by the changes in hormones during the menstrual cycle.

   C It is caused by endometrial tissue growing in areas of the body other than the uterus.

   D It is caused by an infection in the female reproductive system.

6. What is the name of the diagnostic procedure which involves inserting a camera into the abdominal cavity to look for signs of endometriosis? (1)

7. State two methods used to remove tissues affected by endometriosis during surgery. (2)

8. Fill the gaps: _____ medicines and contraceptives control the amount of hormones in the body. This can cause the endometrium tissue to be _____ which will cause less pain. (2)

9. State three signs and symptoms of testicular cancer. (3)

10. What is the name of the surgery where one or more testicles are removed? (1)

11. Fill in the gaps: If both testicles are removed to treat the cancer they will no longer be able to have _____ or make _____. (2)

12. Which is **incorrect** about increased risk of developing testicular cancer? (1)

    A Having a genetic predisposition for the disease

    B Having had undescended testicles

    C Being overweight

    D Having previously been treated with radiotherapy.

13. Outline the role of the cervix in the female reproductive system. (4)

14. Describe the stages of the menstrual cycle (4)

15. Explain the action of hormones in the menopause (4)

16. Describe the use of a laparoscopy for patients with endometriosis. (4)

17. Discuss the benefits and limitations of using a hysterectomy as a treatment for endometriosis. (6)

18. Analyse factors that increase the risk of developing testicular cancer. (6)

www.ingramcontent.com/pod-product-compliance
Lightning Source LLC
Chambersburg PA
CBHW081103070526
44584CB00021B/3182